CRYSTAL Healing Secrets

CRYSTAL Healing Secrets

▲▲▲

Enhance Your Relationships, Sexuality,
Prosperity, and Health

Brett Bravo

WARNER BOOKS

A Time Warner Company

Copyright © 1988 Brett Bravo
All rights reserved.
Warner Books, Inc., 1271 Avenue of the Americas, New York, NY 10020

W A Time Warner Company

Printed in the United States of America
First Printing: May 1988
10 9 8 7 6 5

Cover photo by Al Francekovich

Designed by Giorgetta Bell McRee

Library of Congress Cataloging-in-Publication Data

Bravo, Brett.
  Crystal healing secrets: enhance your relationships, sexuality, prosperity, and health / Brett Bravo.
    p.   cm.
  1. Crystals—Therapeutic use.   I. Title.
RZ415.B72   1988
133—dc19
    ISBN 0-446-38789-4 (pbk.) (U.S.A.)

                                                    88-4212
                                                    CIP

This book is dedicated to:
My mother, Pauline Coleman, who taught me:
"You can do *anything,* if you want to
do it badly enough."

And to:
My daughter, LeSanne Lindborg, who really
believes I can do anything

And to:
Those on other levels of existence who
help me—when I let them.

CONTENTS

ACKNOWLEDGMENTS ix
FOREWORD xi
PROLOGUE xvii

Part One/THE SEARCH FOR THE MIRACULOUS 1

1 Every Miracle Begins as a Search for the Invisible 3
2 Cosmic Crystal Connection: Gems and the Planets.......... 14
3 Religious History of Healing Crystals 22
4 The Coming of the New Age 32

Part Two/UNLOCKING THE CRYSTAL SECRETS 39

5 Choosing Your Crystal 41
6 Twenty-Eight Days to a Miracle: Seven-Minute Healing
   Meditations... 50
7 Understanding the Yin-Yang Principle: Enhancing Sexuality with
   the Love Crystals.. 63
8 Healthy Animals and Plants 75

Part Three/THE HEALING COLOR CONNECTION:
CRYSTALS AND THE PLANETS 81

BIBLIOGRAPHY.. 277

ACKNOWLEDGMENTS

Behind every successful endeavor there is a woman saying, "You can do it!" That has been my experience. Nicki Monaco-Clark was the catalyst for the ingredients of this book. Nicki was born when the Sun was traveling through the constellation of Sagittarius, which causes her to be astrologically known as a fire sign. Fire sign people (Aries, Leo, Sagittarius) have the kind of spirit that demands action!

When Nicki came into my life, I had been attempting to edit my research for another publisher and was really discouraged. She read the material, which lit her fires, and the rest is history! Nicki was the perfect person at the perfect time. She has worked tirelessly and devoted countless hours on her own initiative to edit, rewrite, and manage the production of the final manuscript.

Nicki was the communicator between my agent and publisher. She discovered the planet photos, and she was the one who kept the fires burning over the many months of negotiations with the new publisher.

In the beginning, Nicki did the most perfect thing: she chose a crystal for herself. With a superconscious knowing she chose a pendant of green Malachite. She had not read the chapter on that stone and did not consciously know that it would promote patience! Fire signs are rather short on this virtue. Her patience with the project and me was only matched by her determination to see the physical materialization of this work.

I thank you, we all thank you, Nicki.

I also wish to thank Carla Trader (another fire sign, Leo) who typed the original research papers and spurred me to finish by showing up two hours before I was ready to work every morning for months!

I asked Carla to wear my favorite carved Amethyst neckpiece for two reasons: to clarify thinking and communication, and because she had been on a kidney dialysis machine for fifteen years. This year she had a successful kidney transplant. Thank you, Amethyst. Thank you, Carla.

Thank you John Brockman and Katinka Matson, my agents in New York.

Last, but not least, thanks Elaine Wright, for understanding the meaning of the word deadline.

FOREWORD

I am a scientist and a practitioner with a Ph.D. in clinical psychology. As a scientist I was taught to be interested in truth, facts—what I can measure and, especially, replicate. Most important *is* what I can present to my scientific colleagues that they can replicate. This is significantly limiting. For example, it is emphasized that as scientists we don't examine such things as the soul or anything that we cannot present in measurable terms. *Metaphysics* means "beyond the physical," and so science as science closed the door on scientific investigation of such phenomena until recently. Now, more and more investigators are willing to delve into the areas previously denied. I believe that this is so because we are moving closer to the new Age of Aquarius.

A few brave individuals, willing to face the scoffing, ridicule, and scorn of many fellow scientists, have gone forward. For his scientific research with crystals, we are forever indebted to the genius of Marcel Vogel, working with Quartz crystals at IBM for twenty-five years. To Brett Bravo we are indebted for her pragmatic exploration of the use of crystals in healing physical and emotional disorders and her courage in her willingness to present her work to all of the local and national media. Brett has made it easier for the rest of us to "come out of the closet" with our work in other metaphysical areas.

As a practitioner, I am concerned with what works; and my only limitation is that what I use for healing be ethical and moral. I have been using crystals as a way into meditation and healing since I met Brett. First for myself, and when I was satisfied with the results, for selected patients (those that I believed would not think me "mad").

I met Brett about five years ago. I was going through a rough time of my life, dealing with the depression associated with a marriage I knew I couldn't continue. The issues for me were old ones that I had dealt with many times over the years in thousands of sessions of psychoanalysis and group therapy to no avail. I was not in the least metaphysical at the time. While browsing in a bookstore, I came upon a display of business cards advertising all kinds of psychic and spiritual help. Out of curiosity (and despair) I asked the woman behind the counter to recommend someone to me for help. She sent me to Brett.

By the end of my session with Brett, I knew more about my problem areas than I believed was possible in one session. She recommended that I meditate with an Amethyst crystal. She had me choose one from a tray of such uncut natural gems. It was mine to keep and carry with me. She gave me an instruction sheet to go with it and led me through my first treatment. I felt no different but was determined to give it a try since I was told a breakthrough could occur within one week and significant changes within twenty-one days. To be honest, I felt desperate enough to try anything no matter how skeptical I was about her concepts.

In a few days I found that I was experiencing the relationship with my wife in a very different way, and that which I had been holding in was being expressed. My wife was who she was and that's the way it was to be with her. As I contemplated a divorce, since months of marriage therapy wasn't helping, Brett gave me a Sapphire to work with. I felt my depression lifting, a peacefulness about my choice, and best of all, I wasn't ruminating about our disagreements as I had been. Over a period of several months, Brett instructed me in the use of a series of crystals, each helping me through a particular period.

It was a whole new beginning for me as I felt, and was, better with each passing day. I knew I had to investigate this for myself in as scientific a way as possible. Brett became my teacher. She gave me books to read and loaned me crystals to try on myself and my psychotherapy patients. In a short while, there was no doubt in my mind I had a most powerful healing tool.

From the study and work with crystals it was a short distance into the investigation of the occult, metaphysics, spiritual—call it what you wish. There were truths I never knew existed about life, spirit, soul, God, the cosmos, ad infinitum. My studies and my growth, human and Divine, led me to many teachers and teachings. And finally, to the truth Brett told me in my beginnings: "There will come a time when your teacher will be your own Highest Self." I do believe I had the courage to present my research findings on "past lives" at a national convention of the American Psychological Association because of Brett as my first metaphysics mentor and, especially, her courage.

In my wildest human fantasies I would never have believed that from a single Amethyst crystal an institute could grow.

I still wear that first Amethyst given to me by Brett. You were guided here as she was guided to write this for you. Certainly we are of One Entity with Everything in Creation. What We Know You Know and what You Know We Know. We merely have to remember that We Know It. May you bring Light to Yourself.

With Peace, Light, and Love,

Lawrence Vogel, Ph.D.
The Joshua Institute of Light
Solana Beach, California
November 18, 1987

"Both shamans and scientists personally pursue research into the mysteries of the Universe. Both believe that the underlying causal processes of that Universe are hidden from ordinary view. Neither master shamans nor master scientists allow the dogma of ecclesiastical and political authorities to interfere with their explorations. It was no accident that Galileo was accused of witchcraft (shamanism)."

—Michael Harner
("The Way of the Shaman")
Chairman, Anthropology Section
New York Academy of Sciences, 1982

PROLOGUE

"It is through elevating and transcending our perceptions of space . . . time . . . energy . . . matter . . . consciousness, and acting in accordance with the Universe that true healing of ourselves occurs."

—**Tai Chi Chuan**

▲▲▲

Let's face it . . . I have a bias. My work is based on my own personal philosophy.

. . . I believe in a Designing Force.

. . . I believe the Universe is a safe place to be.

. . . I believe the planets revolving in their cycles are transmitting cosmic rays to each other and to the Earth in a pattern set up by the Designing Force to aid all beings in their evolutionary growth and that other cosmic rays from unknown sources also affect human life.

. . . I believe all beings are striving to grow and evolve in an upward and forward direction to ultimately learn creativity in the capacity of the Designing Force.

. . . I believe the Earth level to be the most gross and

basic physical level in the Universe, and therefore the beginning level on a par with kindergarten.

. . . I believe Earth to be a school in which we experience progressive lives (reincarnation) that include every experience possible on the physical level in order to understand and truly know this gross level of manifestation.

. . . I believe there are innumerable levels of consciousness and that Earthlings can reach levels that are not physical, such as mental and spiritual levels.

WE CAN HAVE MENTAL CONTROL OVER OUR PHYSICAL BODIES.

WE CAN HAVE SPIRITUAL CONTROL OVER OUR MENTAL-EMOTIONAL BODIES.

. . . I believe each person on Earth to be totally responsible for all circumstances of birth and able to choose to act from free will at all times.

. . . I believe in order to create our own bodies we must experience all the experiments that do not get the desired results, such as genetic defects.

. . . I believe we have set up physical situations for ourselves wherein we automatically create psychological learning experiences. Ghetto living can create anger, rebellion, and crime, which can create incarceration—or it can be overcome. Everything depends on the individual.

. . . I believe as we become more highly evolved after numerous lifetimes, we become more in tune with the nonphysical levels of manifestation. We develop the invisible bodies: Mental, Emotional, and Spiritual. The right and left brain become integrated. Logic and intuition, male and female polarities, operate more closely in tandem.

. . . I believe there is consciousness in everything in the physical world. Molecular structure designates vibration . . . vibration designates life . . . life designates some form of consciousness.

. . . I believe the Designing Force has given every living thing an action and a reason to interact with every other living thing.

. . . I believe that there is no death, only transformation, recycling, and evolution of everything in the Universe.

With this personal belief system of mine in mind, I invite each of you merely to consider the possibilities that I now describe, concerning the interaction of cosmic rays, Earth crystals, and the physical and invisible bodies of the human.

Part One

THE SEARCH FOR THE MIRACULOUS

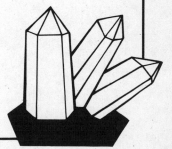

1/ Every Miracle Begins as a Search for the Invisible

I am a metaphysician. I don't think most people know what in the world that word means. *Meta* means "beyond," so *metaphysical* means "beyond the physical." When you say "metaphysician," people have a tendency to think you're talking about being a doctor, and I'm talking about that too.

I have an urgent need to make people feel better. I'm concerned about how people feel, and I'm concerned with showing them how to take their own power to make themselves feel better. In this book I'm going to teach you to do the same things successfully to make yourself well. But not just on the physical level, because I don't believe we're ill just on the physical level.

3

I believe that there are bodies that are invisible in addition to the physical body. There are three: the Spiritual, Mental, and Emotional. You will notice that I have capitalized the separate bodies because they are very special and you should think of these parts of yourself as very special. The Spirit Body gives us life. The Spirit Body has to do with the heart because that's where the spirit lives. The Mental Body makes our conscious brain work. That's where the Mental Body lives, in the conscious, subconscious, and superconscious parts of the brain. The Emotional Body surrounds the physical body and is larger than even the Mental Body because we can project our emotions. People can sense how we feel when we walk in the door. They don't recognize that. They don't realize how much we respond to what is unsaid and unseen in our lives. That's what "meta" means.

The Spirit Body in the heart is like a fuse box in a house with lots of wiring in it that goes all over the body. It is the current that gives the body life. There's another fuse box in the brain that gives the Mental Body life. You know the Mental Body dies even when the Spirit Body still lives because there are people all over the world on life-support systems. Their Mental Body is dead but their physical body still lives. There is the Emotional Body operating out of the solar plexus where another fuse box contains separate circuitry. There are those whose Emotional Bodies are dead even though their physical bodies still live who are in asylums and back rooms. Their Emotional Body is either partially or totally dead while their other two bodies, the Physical and Mental, are still alive.

So I treat the different bodies of a person. When a client comes to me for a reading, even though I may not have met them previously, I will be led to choose a specific type of background music, which begins to affect their Emotional Body. I serve them a glass of water in which I have placed the lithium-based Lapidolite crystal, a natural mood balancer affecting the Mental Body. There are color vibrations in furniture coverings and paintings that affect the Spirit Body. This combination causes a response that is noticeable in the physical body. It is very common for my clients to say within a very few moments that they are feeling better. Needless to say, the whole environment is also affected by the crystal specimens placed everywhere in view.

At this point the client is in a relaxed and secure mood. I hand them my tray of special healing crystals and ask them to handle each crystal, to study each, and give the crystal time to interact with their electromagnetic field. I ask the client to choose one crystal to hold throughout their consultation. The client may ask me, "How shall I know which one to choose?" I explain, "Choose the one you like the best." When I observe the crystal that the client has chosen, it helps me to know in which of the bodies they are searching for balance.

The healing that's been going on for thousands of years has been treating only the physical body. With Freud, we started to treat the Mental and Emotional Bodies a little bit. And of course, the church has always tried to treat the Spirit Body. I am attempting to reach all three bodies so the physical body will respond and be healthy. That's what being a metaphysician is all about . . . healing the unseen bodies that have manifested physical dis-ease.

My focus is on healing the invisible bodies. My belief, based on years of personal studies of physical illnesses, "accidents," allergies, and surgeries, is that the physical body responds to mental, emotional, or spiritual imbalance. Even the medical profession has come to the conclusion that a very large percentage of their patients' complaints are brought about by psychosomatic mis-understanding.

The following is a simple example of how our body will

speak out for us in the form of illness when we don't speak out literally about how we think (Mental Body) or how we feel (Emotional Body).

I met a new client shortly after a recent surgery, in which a tumor, larger than a volleyball, was removed from her abdomen. This woman had complained for years to her physicians that something was wrong with her. She had been treated with tranquilizers and diagnosed as psychosomatic, functioning under too much stress. Both the woman and her physicians were actually correct.

Her stress was caused by a belief that she could not speak her mind. For years she had withheld her feelings, believing they would bring her punishment or abandonment if she expressed them. These feelings were shoved down inside of her abdomen and held in a collection of actual physical mass. By refusing to speak, her physical body had to speak for her.

All of this drama can be eliminated from our lives when we begin to deal with our invisible bodies. It is possible that the woman's tumor could have been reduced without dangerous life-threatening surgery if a competent counselor, skilled in the use of visualization, had been sought out earlier in her treatment. The ideal remedy would have been to use a crystal in active exercises that would have opened communication and balanced the invisible bodies.

Her tumor was the result of an imbalance in the Emotional Body that could have been affected by: a) wearing and meditating with a Pink Tourmaline for emotional expression; b) wearing and meditating with an Amethyst to bring clarity and purity of thought to the Mental Body; c) wearing and meditating with a Rose Quartz for soft and gentle love of the self (Spirit Body) and others; d) wearing and meditating with an Emerald, working on the Mental Body, which causes a "coming clean" with the truth of what is real and not imagined.

When we began working together, she chose, through her own superconscious knowing, an Emerald, to come clean with the truth. She is now preventing further physical complications by using the crystal vibration to aid in her self healing.

Now, you may be asking me, "How does this crystal vibration work on the invisible bodies?" The electromagnetic fields (rate of vibration) or frequencies of crystals and certain colored stones can aid us in harmonizing our own electromagnetic fields through the "tuning fork effect." Let's imagine two people holding matched tuning forks. The first person strikes theirs so that it begins to vibrate at a certain frequency or pitch. The second person is still holding theirs without striking it, and yet it begins to vibrate at the same frequency! Now, why is this? This occurs through transmission of atoms from one similarly tuned object to another one, finely tuned to the same rate of vibration. When this occurs, they are able to sing in harmony! In this model the crystal or gemstone is the first tuning fork and transmits its vibration to the human being as the receiving tuning fork that begins to vibrate at the same frequency as the crystal. This is the healing/harmonizing effect!

Add to this innate intelligence of the body to harmonize, the ability to transmit *thought* through the crystal in order to amplify the healing/harmonizing effect, and you have the power to heal yourself! Crystals are transmitters of cosmic rays. When we send our intentions through the crystal and ask it to aid us in getting our desired results, the vibration of that thought is amplified, bringing it nearer its physical manifestation.

There are still people who may think that crystals are far-out, maybe more related to the dark side, which makes them afraid. Well, I can understand how they might think something like that. It's only because they're not thinking it through. What they really need to do is to get to the bottom line and ask, "Who made the crystals? Why are they on the Earth?"

Crystals are a product of nature, like a tree. Why is a tree on Earth? For one thing, trees are beautiful and everyone loves them. For another, they have leaves that clean the air and manufacture oxygen. And, because we can cut them up and make lumber out of them with which to build things. Real simple. But we didn't find that out right away. It took millions of years before we figured it out. And just because we cut a tree up and make lumber out of it to build something doesn't mean we are doing witchcraft. But we are taking matters into our own hands. We're taking something that was there for us and we're using it.

Coal is created in the same process of nature as crystals. Both are made by the cycles of the earth—namely heat, pressure, and time. Coal and oil run our factories, fuel our automobiles, and heat our homes. They've been there all the time. Crystals provide a form of energy that we are just beginning to explore.

The idea of crystal energy is no more strange than the idea of electricity must have been in Ben Franklin's day. We have only recently discovered electricity, X rays, and radio waves. Each of these energies was present in the space around humans, penetrating our bodies, filling the air we breathe, the water we drink, and indirectly keeping us in a state of support. Eventually when their "secrets" were uncovered by our scientists, we were able to expand their value to us as diagnostic and healing or solving energies.

Scientists realize that the human body has electrical currents that can be complemented by scientifically harnessed electricity in knitting broken bones. Captured X rays make possible vision into the heretofore hidden areas of the body. Radioactive rays are focused to kill unwanted misbehaving cells that kill our healthy cells in cancerous growths. Every miracle begins as a search for the invisible.

I first became involved in the crystals when I moved from the Northwest to Southern California, where the change in intellectual climate freed me from a lifetime of psychic restriction. (I believe certain crystal veins found in the earth have caused a different vibration here, which stimulates healing open-mindedness.) I had graduated from college as an interior designer after completing extensive research with a disciple of Dr. Max Lüscher, the prominent Swiss psychologist who pioneered the first studies on the psychology of color and its effects on people's minds and bodies. I used that education for twenty years as a professional interior designer. I used my knowledge of color and light to create health and happiness in environments. In 1976 I returned to college to take another degree in psychological counseling and changed careers.

In Southern California I joined a group who were conducting a psychic energy experiment. We met one hour weekly to focus our minds toward the Source of all energy. Our object was to multiply the energy and return it to Earth in whatever area would be most beneficial to all.

At the first sending, I experienced a trance state and an out-of-body experience in which I verbally related information concerning seven gem crystals that were specifically suggested for each member of the group.

When I returned to my normal state, I was amazed by the information I had received. I had no previous conscious knowledge of gems or crystals. The information continued to flow through me for short periods at each weekly gathering.

At first, I didn't trust it. I said, "I have to prove this to my logical left brain." I began to do serious study on the actual mineral elements and/or metals present in crystals that cause the very specific frequencies in each colored gem. I studied gemology and mineralogy. As friends began to notice my changing focus, I received clippings and materials to read on the subject from many areas around the world. One of my most prized possessions is an original copy of Dana's *System of Minerology*, updated to 1899. The author, James Dwight Dana, was professor of physics and curator of the mineral collection at Yale University.

I discovered that a world-renowned expert, John Sinkankas, lived here in Southern California and had published in 1964 the most up-to-date book on crystallography, called *Mineralogy for Amateurs*.

These two books became my bibles, along with every other book I could find for sale with any reference whatsoever to rocks, gems, crystals, or minerals. Most of these books were not concerned with spiritual, esoteric, or healing remedies. A few of them contained historical references to ancient manuscripts that intrigued me. I kept thinking about the ancient manuscripts and the references to gem crystals in the Bible. It just became imperative to me to search them out.

Like a miracle, I was offered a position as an agent for a portrait artist that would take me to several countries. I did not realize at that time how important it is to get a clear picture of what we want. As I look back over my life, I realize that nothing ever happens in our lives until we decide what we really *want* to happen. My clarity had attracted the opportunity.

I took the job, sublet my apartment, and not knowing exactly why or how, began a year and a half tracing the historical uses of gem crystals in the libraries and museums of Europe and the U.S.

I visited every natural history display in all of the major cities in the U.S. The Smithsonian in Washington, D.C., is of course the grandest and most complete. The most exciting experience was the three months in Rome, perusing the Vatican Treasury and library of ancient manuscripts.

My travels included Athens, the island of Rhodes, Spain, all the historic cities in Italy, Austria, Germany, and Great Britain. I returned with nine extra pieces of luggage! I had to do a lot of fast talking at Air France in Paris to bring home my books and research papers.

I also began to experiment with the crystals on my own physical, Mental, Spirit, and Emotional Bodies. I was attracted to the Amethyst. I always liked the color, and being around that crystal made me feel really good, even though I had always thought that I *should* like my Sapphire "birth stone." By this time in my research, I had discovered twelve separate birth-stone lists and translations that contained diverse information. I decided to keep an Amethyst nearby while I was researching. I noticed more clarity of thought. My friends noticed better communication. I became dedicated to using the Amethyst on my body by holding it over the three centers every day. I carried it in my clothing, slept with it, and even bathed with it. And I took careful daily notes on my responses to it. The bottom-line result on my physical body was the complete cessation of what I considered to be the normal amount of colds and respiratory complaints.

After using the crystals I describe in this book, and taking notes on the effect they had on me, I really experienced a dose of self-consciousness. I became totally aware of what my individual bodies were doing and the results they had on my physical body.

I began to realize there were metaphysical reasons why humanity had chosen certain acupuncture points on the body to cover with jewelry. At this point I experimented with symbols and shapes to add to, or mount, the crystals into rings, bracelets, pendants, tie clips, or bolo ties for men, women, and children.

Whether the crystal is natural or faceted seems to have no apparent bearing on the process. The Hindus believed the clarity of the crystal made it more powerful, but I have not found this to be so. The clarity certainly makes the faceted gem crystal more expensive and unavailable to the average client. For that reason I generally suggest a natural, uncut crystal.

I believe that each person has a superconscious knowing of which crystal is best for them. If one of my clients can have access to view and touch a sample of each of the crystals I use, most choose perfectly for themselves.

I suggest the crystal chosen be kept on the body at all times, worn preferably at the heart chakra on a long chain or at the throat chakra. "Chakra" is the word that is used to designate the power centers of the body by Hindu yogis and others. In the Oriental way of healing using acupuncture, these chakras are taken into the complete electrical systems of the body and are called meridians. The heart, solar plexus, and throat chakras appear to be the most effective of the seven chakras, or power centers, of the body, where Universal energy is received.

In the beginning of my work with clients, I would wrap or cap the crystal in gold or silver so it could be easily attached to a chain. Gold and silver are both crystals, too. The Sun's vibrations are transmitted by the gold, masculine, crystal, and the Moon's rays are transmitted by the silver, feminine, crystal. Using both silver and gold together within the same piece creates a more perfect yin-yang, masculine-feminine, balance.

As a result of my study, using the Amethyst as an aid to my thinking, I believe I've become a better communicator. This book is a case in point. I have been able to say more concisely what I want people to understand. The Amethyst rules communicaton. I wear it at my throat, the communications center, where these vibrations emerge into the ethers around us and are picked up by other people.

In the following pages I will explain my understanding of why the crystals work. Parts II and III will explain specific meditations for healing.

The crystal/planetary way of healing presented in this book should not be considered an exclusive method of confronting medical problems. It should be viewed as an adjunct to orthodox medical or psychological treatment, unless contrary medical advice is given.

In some cases the rebalancing of the mind, body, and spirit that is necessary may cause physical symptoms or emotional amplification that feels like distress. This is natural. I always caution my clients to persevere as the eventual relief is welcome compensation.

I also stress that the crystal must not become a placebo. The cure is centered within the mind of the client, not within the crystal. As in all healing practices, the prescription is doubly effective if the client takes responsibility and cooperates for their own best interest.

2/Cosmic Crystal Connection: Gems and the Planets

"All particles are created from energy and vanish into energy. The whole universe appears as a dynamic web of inseparable energy patterns."

—**Fritjof Capra,** physicist
The Tao of Physics

▲▲▲

EARTH'S HEALING ENERGIES

Our Mother is the Earth, our bodies came from hers, in that we are made of the elements from her body. You know that we have calcium in bones, teeth, and nails, iron in our blood, and countless other metals, phosphates, and crystal salts. The plants that we eat all extract these elements from Mother Earth and we extract them from the

14

plants. We constantly circulate, recycle, and transform the energies from our Mother.

She must also have a source of power and sustenance in order to continue to nurture us. Where does it come from? Since she is a cell in the body of the Universe swimming in the Universal bloodstream that we call space, she must be extracting her "vitamins" from the Sun and other powerful planets around her. How could her body be like ours? It seems very possible that she could have a physical working system like ours with a network of nerves, veins, capillaries, and acupuncture points along electrical meridians. (Science has proven that we are electrical.)

If this is so, then the veins of crystals, which include gold, silver, and other metals as well as Quartz and gem crystals, that are found throughout her body are an important part of her nurturing system.

Just as she continually recreates coal, oil, and gases to give us mechanical energies, she also produces crystals to give us healing energies. She regularly brings them closer to the surface by tectonic shifting and volcanic activity. Her body processes are very similar to ours, and she tends to us as we do our children.

In our Universal body, Earth is also sending a type of Earth-ray to the other planets. As this vibration comes up from her center, its healing energy fills our bodies. It is an electromagnetic field that can be captured in her crystal veins. When we harvest the crystals and use them in healing, we mix their electro-bionic-magnetic frequencies into our own. We are in actuality treating the auras or invisible bodies that our brain, solar plexus, and heart are radiating out around us. This is taken in by the physical body and our energies are *CHANGED*.

When you begin working with your own crystal, you will begin to allow the Earth's healing energy to be focused on you. Your physical body will respond.

But the crystals reflect more than just the Earth's healing

energy. They also reflect the healing rays of the Universe.

The Sun, Moon, Mercury, Mars, Venus, Jupiter, Saturn, Uranus, Neptune, and Pluto are transmitting signals, tones, or vibrations that have been picked up clearly since our space probes began monitoring. When we hear the terms X ray, ultraviolet ray, infrared, etc., do we think of these as invisible energy? Do we realize that these rays are coming to Earth from somewhere "out there"? Even our most common source of energy is invisible electricity.

These cosmic rays are feeding our Mother Earth, penetrating deeply into her body, activating her heart, and circulating her healing energies through the network of crystal veins.

Marsha Adams, a biologist conducting experiments at the Stanford University Medical School for over ten years, has hypothesized that the phenomena of changes in the geomagnetic field of the Earth cause changes in biological and psychological processes in the inhabitants.

Her work includes evidence that laboratory experiments on animals is very definitely influenced by times of geophysical differences. She has also had astonishing success at predicting earthquakes by monitoring physiological and psychological changes in humans.

This is but a small account of many scientific references to actual invisible influences on physical life by Mother Earth.

To understand the role of the planets in healing, we can look to the ancient art of astrology. In ancient religious manuscripts of the oldest religions on Earth, astrologers wrote about the movements of planets that were not even visible. As far as we know, they had no telescopes. Today, with all our technology, we see that their calculations were accurate to an astonishing degree.

Astrology teaches that the cycles of the moving planets cause seasons and cycles on Earth. It further claims that the planets release invisible waves of energy that affect the Earth, from the tides to our own personalities.

The planets were in a certain celestial configuration when we were born. Our new bodies received rays, waves, and vibrations immediately upon drawing our first breaths. That was our first intake of Cosmic Current. At that moment we received a very individual imprint and impression of vibration.

The current of the Cosmos can be compared to the bloodstream of the human body. It is the energy force that includes all the scientifically described energies that interact to create magnetism and gravity. Cosmic Current repels and attracts all the planets and stars in each solar system so that they move in space consistently without colliding or straying out of their prescribed patterns. This current carries the specific vibrations from each planet and star to every other planet and star in each solar system, and from each solar system and universe to every other solar system and universe.

Astrologers and even now astronomers are aware that these signals or vibrations or waves or particles are experienced as invisible rays of energy by us, the recipients of the Cosmic Current.

The more highly evolved gems and minerals are simply receivers of these specific planetary rays. Because of the mathematical makeup of the Universe, the geometric structure of the gems allows certain waves or rays to pass through them and others to be absorbed or trapped inside. This causes the molecules of the gem to vibrate at a rate directed by the rays of a certain planet, and gives it color.

The mathematical nature of the Universe is observed by physicists such as Albert Einstein in that all phenomena can be written into a mathematical equation. For an elementary example, an ear of corn always contains thirteen rows. Pinecones and simple daisies also exhibit consistent numbers of rows. Throughout the Earth and Universe we measure with mathematics the orbits of everything and find them mathematically consistent. The Moon is in a twenty-eight-day cycle and our Sun is in a 365-day cycle.

Astrologers tell us when the Moon, Sun, and planets are in a measurable geometric position or equation to send their vibrations to Earth, which will have a specific effect on certain individuals.

Each gem contains elements that reflect or absorb light waves. Light waves are vibrations that come to Earth from many sources. We know the Sun to be our main source of light. All the other planets are so far away we cannot imagine that their energy waves could be strong enough to reach Earth with any intensity. Although space exploration has proven that the planets do transmit impulses, we do not know the scientific power of most of the planets.

Deep in a bunker in Minnesota, scientists are observing cosmic rays that surge through the atmosphere with 10^{17} volts of energy—200,000 times more energy than has ever been produced in a laboratory and far greater than energy levels of most cosmic rays.

The high-energy cosmic rays were detected by researchers who were conducting experiments in a laboratory buried 2,000 feet beneath solid rock. The newly discovered rays follow a straight path all the way down through the Earth's crust.

University of Minnesota physicist Marvin Marshak, a member of the research team, told Geo Magazine *that "I and my colleagues do not know where the cosmic rays originate or what produces them."*

—*Geo Magazine, Vol. 5*
September 1983

The Earth's crust is composed of over two thousand identified minerals. If the energy wave of a certain planet is received by Earth, it is possible that the basic mineral of that planet, which is on Earth in the form of a crystal, would pick up and relay the vibration. If we are influenced physically and psychically by planetary emissions, having the crystal related to the important planet or planets would magnify the process.

Each of the signs of the zodiac is assigned a ruling planet. Each person receives vibrations for specific reasons from a specific planet. Each planet is also broadcasting through a specific gem-crystal or groups of gems of similar color.

Planets transmitting the silver and white ray through Diamond, Clear Quartz, Agate, Opal, and Pearl are a total of all our Solar System, including stars and unknown originators of planetary rays. The effects are felt as divine guidance, cosmic consciousness, balance, and particularly in the case of the Opal, psychic awareness.

The planet transmitting the red ray through the Rose Quartz, Carnelian, Garnet, Ruby, Coral, and Fire Opal is Mars. It brings zest for life, self-love, energy-passion, self-remembering, and in the case of the Coral, willingness to cooperate. The planet Pluto transmits the dark-red burgundy ray through Garnet and Sugilite.

The planet transmitting the blue ray through the Blue Topaz, Lapis Lazuli, Sapphire, and Turquoise is Uranus. The effects are felt as protection, calmness, release from sadness, alertness, and visualization of perfect health.

The planet that is transmitting a blue/pink ray (which is not visible to our sight in our light spectrum) is Venus. It vibrates the Aquamarine, which brings peace of mind.

The planet that is transmitting the green ray through Chrysoprase, Emerald, Green Garnets, Jade, Malachite, and Peridot is Saturn. Its effect on us is to bring control of appetites, honesty, problem solving, patience, and spiritual understanding.

The planet transmitting the Violet ray through Kunzite, Amethyst, and Sugilite is Mercury. The Kunzite also transmits the light blue/pink ray from Venus. This violet ray brings clarity and purity of thought and communication. In the case of Sugilite (which also transmits the burgundy ray from Pluto) it brings a deep, primordial recollection of other primitive but intelligent states of being that we have experienced. It brings the deep understanding of how death transforms into birth. With Kunzite it brings the knowledge of unconditional love from the Universe.

The planet transmitting the yellow ray through the Golden Topaz and Tiger's-eye is Jupiter. The brown ray from an unknown source is also transmitting through Tiger's-eye. The Topaz brings joy, abundance, awareness of the present moment, and optimism. The Tiger's-eye brings concentration and energy focus.

Each one of the crystals affects different invisible bodies so that the physical body responds toward healing itself of ailments or complaints connected to mental, emotional, or spiritual imbalance.

When the ancient lists were translated from the Sanskrit, they ascribed certain gems to the seven known planets. We now recognize ten, including our Moon and Sun. Uranus, Pluto, and Neptune all moved into our area of the galaxy within the last two hundred years. Since there are twelve zodiacal signs, there must be two more planets destined to move into our area of the galaxy. The two signs of the zodiac awaiting new rulers are Virgo and Libra, who are now sharing rulers with Taurus and Gemini.

The discovery of additional planets has also led to a complete corruption of the original birth-stone theory. The modern birth stone is now a myth based on a fact of history.

Many people already know from a knowledge of astrology that their Sun sign on which birth stones are based is sometimes not their most dominant sign anyway. It could be something else in your chart, such as your rising sign, your Moon, some configuration with Saturn. We could use Saturn and its aspects because Saturn is the teacher. Wherever it is in your birth chart and whatever the aspects to it are will tell you what you're working on in this lifetime. Saturn also rules rocks, minerals, and crystals.

3/ Religious History of Healing Crystals

"O thou afflicted, tossed with tempest and not comforted, behold, I will lay thy stones with fair colors and lay the foundations with sapphires. And I will make thy windows of agates and thy gates of carbuncles and all the borders of pleasant stones."

—Isaiah 54:11–12

▲▲▲

The day I was interviewed on the Sally Jessy Raphael show in Macon, Georgia, there were 3,500 Bible Belt Southerners in the audience. I was happy for my Christian background, because I do remember some verses from the Bible and I have done a lot of research at the Vatican as well as libraries all over the world. I know that there's a tremendous amount of information about the crystals in the Bible and that equally large amounts of information have been taken out. I was able to tell the audience that if they believed the Bible strictly on faith, why would they eliminate the crystal information? It comes from the very same book. If people are going to talk about the Bible, they had better go back and read the whole thing, because the oldest treatise on crystals and their miraculous powers has been described in this, the most famous of manuscripts, the Old Testament.

Exodus (28:15–30) describes a religious breastplate worn during ceremonies by Aaron, the first High Priest of Israel. It is said to have had twelve enormous gems, three placed horizontally with another three rows underneath. Each gem was inscribed with the name of one of the twelve tribes of Israel. Each also had mysterious powers that could be used by the priests in divining matters of law, religion, war, and healing. I find it exciting and in many ways very plausible to speculate that this may actually have been a highly technical computer or inter-galactic communication device.

A Samaritan version of the Book of Joshua also carried an account of the breastplate. From these writings, a biblical historian observed in 1833 that probably after the capture of Jerusalem by the Roman Emperor Titus, A.D. 70, the treasures of the temple were carried off to Rome where they were deposited in the Temple of Concord. During the sacking of Rome by the Vandals, A.D. 455, the breastplate may have been hidden with other treasures.

A historian living during the time the Vandals triumphed in Persia stated that the "Vessels of the Jews" were carried through the streets of Constantinople A.D. 534. Although researchers have tried to trace the fate of the sacred jewels, it is thought they may still be buried in some unknown treasure chamber in one of the old Persian capitals.

The stones as we know them today have different names. The primary stone in the breastplate, however, is believed to have been a Ruby. *Les Lapidaires Français* states that the

Ruby was the "gem of gems" that God commanded be placed around the neck of Aaron.

The description of the breastplate in Hebrew tradition was held in high regard by the Jews of that era. Thousands of years later, after the crucifixion of Christ, St. John the Apostle described in the New Testament Book of Revelation (21:9–21) his dream of a "New Jerusalem" as it would appear in the future. "And the foundations of the walls of the city were garnished with all manner of precious stones," he wrote.

Each gem represented a quality of life. We cannot know for certain what John's symbology was, but in later rabbinical writings, for instance, Tiger's-eye was thought to designate justice, Sapphire, the light of celestial hope, and Jasper, the truth of faith.

The city of the future was pictured by St. John as descending from the sky and having twelve gates of entry. Each gate was a single Pearl. From this writing we derive the expression "the pearly gates of heaven."

Rabanus Maurus, Archbishop of Mainz, translated the passages in Revelation, A.D. 786, so each gem corresponded to one of the twelve Apostles. In his interpretation, Tiger's-eye was the symbol of St. James, known for his generous nature. The gem represented James' inner charity. The Archbishop's treatise also attributed Chrysoprase as a demonstration of the blessed martyrs and their reward.

Writing in the last half of the tenth century, Andreas, Bishop of Caesarea, researched the Book of Revelation. His list of Apostolic gems derived from St. John's vision included the Amethyst, listed as the twelfth layer of the city's foundation, and designated to represent the Apostle Matthias, chosen to replace Judas.

The order in which the foundation of New Jerusalem was delineated also determined the way in which stones were attributed to the months of the year. The place the

Apostles occupied within the stone layers of the metaphorical city influenced this development as well.

However, many theologians felt that only Christ should be regarded as the foundation of His church. Consequently, the symbolism of the stones was made to apply to Christ alone.

The Hindu and Buddhist religions contain many ancient writings that are similar in tone and subject to the Hebrew Old Testament. It is of special interest to speculate on their origins. Continuing study on these translations using newly discovered archaeological clues is enlightening today's scholars.

The Hindu Puranas describe a wonderful jeweled city called Dwaraka, decorated with Pearls and other precious gems, where the Lord Krishna received his visitors. The Buddhist glorious royal city of Kusavati described in Mah Sudassava Scittareta parallels the Christian Book of Revelation in its descriptions of gates of Jade and ramparts of Coral.

In every religion found on Earth, jewels are mentioned as significant to esoteric mysteries. There are references made to precious stones in the Babylonian Talmud long before Genesis. In the Muhammadan Koran gems are described in spiritual rituals. The ancient Egyptians, who lived a very advanced mental life, used gems as an intrinsic part of their spiritual and medicinal ablutions.

After an ancient Hebrew text, The Book of Raziel, received a Greco-Roman translation, myth and legend intertwined. The Book of Wings, as it was called, described the magical purposes of gem engravings.

Both pagans and Christians engraved symbols of the zodiac, Christian lore, and political figures on precious gems. A Topaz with a falcon engraved upon it would assure the owner good relationships with the ruling citizens and lawyers. On a Tiger's-eye, a man with his right arm raised would assure justice. The Sun carved upon Malachite would be used as a protection against enchantments, and a Garnet would guard the wearer from all perils of travel if a lion was engraved on it.

Of course, the original symbology intended for healing use has been lost to us now. Actual engravings upon certain crystals, however, would remind the subconscious of the owner to hasten their own personal healing; they were never intended for universal use. Each person used a gem and a symbol for their own personal healing, much like a medical prescription. You don't give someone else your prescription.

For instance, Amethyst, engraved with the image of a bear, was said to defend the wearer from drunkenness. There are writers today who still attribute this power to the Amethyst, when actually it may have been related to a particular complaint in those days.

By the way, it is thought that the origin of that myth may have to do with Amethyst's being the color of wine. The story also alludes to the legend of Christ at the wedding party, when He turned water into wine. If water is poured into a vessel made of red stone or clay, the water turns to the color of wine but doesn't intoxicate.

There have always been talismans and amulets. Archaeologists, anthropologists, and psychologists studying this phenomena have seen their use as tools. Instinctively we have kept the minerals and gems as our talismans. Evolved and intellectual though we may be, our basic instinct to be one with the planet causes us to keep close contact with gems.

The Christians A.D. 355 discouraged the many beliefs in the powers of gems. The Council of Laodicea decreed that churchmen were to discontinue all use of astrology and amulets. Their purpose was to discourage "pagan" superstitions. Anyone found using them was expelled from the church.

Nevertheless, the clergy retained their own use of precious stones throughout history. In the twelfth century, the Sapphire was favored for use in ecclesiastical rings. Deemed sacred, Sapphire was honored as rendering the wearer better able to hear and understand the most obscure mystery.

Even today in the Roman Catholic Church, a new cardinal receives the red hat and a Sapphire ring bestowed upon him by the Pope, who wears an Amethyst transmitting the violet ray, which is known to be the most healing. The violet flame of St. Germaine, the patron saint of healers, is captured in the Amethyst.

The vessel (called the monstrance) still used by the Catholic church today to hold the sacred host representing the physical body of Christ during the ritual of benediction at the conclusion of High Mass is often surrounded by twelve precious gems, corresponding to the twelve apostles, the twelve tribes of Israel, the twelve gems on the breastplate of Aaron, and the twelve transmitting planets of the sign of the zodiac. The priest may not know, as he holds this instrument in front of his congregation, he is also directing cosmic rays to them.

Reference to the heavenly color of the Sapphire, considered the "bluest of all blues," is made in numerous places within the Old Testament. The sacred nature of the stone was unquestioned in that the law given to Moses is said to have been engraved on the holy tablets in Sapphire. And according to Scriptures, as Moses and the elders worshipped the "God of Israel," they saw under His feet a pavement worked in Sapphire stone. Since there are large deposits of Lapis Lazuli in Afghanistan, this may have been the blue stone. It would be easier to carve as it is a much softer stone.

One of the oldest and possibly the most interesting of the talismanic jewels of Hindu origin is the Naortna, a nine-gem necklace in which each stone corresponds to a planet, the Sun, and the Moon. Its design, set counterclockwise around the Sun, represented by a Ruby, combined powerful astrological influences. The Pearl, considered by the Hindus as one of the five great gems, was placed in the southeast to represent the Moon.

Emeralds are often referred to in the oldest rabbinical legends of the Hebrews. It is related that the Creator gave four precious stones to King Solomon, each representing the four cardinal points. The Emerald was said to quicken the intelligence and to bring about honesty.

During the sixteenth century, a religious relic cut from Emerald was believed to be preserved in Genoa. The "Sacro Catino" was a cup or dish supposed to have been used by Jesus at the Last Supper. When the Church was in dire need of money, it is said the dish was pawned to a wealthy Jew. He had several glass copies made and pawned them to other wealthy lenders, assuring them that the Church would redeem them with interest. Both the original vessel and the "rich Jew of Metz" disappeared.

Again in the Old Testament, there are accounts of a stone in the tent of Abraham that put forth light. Noah was supposed to have a stone on the Ark that lit his way. There are so many legends about the luminosity of certain precious stones that it is quite simple to agree that legend is based on fact. There must have been a time when the gems we know today were used in a different way, perhaps in conjunction with each other, causing them to light up.

The fourteenth century had many religious manuscripts concerning gems—even though the Catholic church had denied parishioners their use long before. During the Dark Ages, that sorry time in history, the Church decreed to the masses that they must bring to the altar all their precious jewels to be cleansed and blessed. A special mass was written to rid them of their evil. The gems were never returned to their owners, and the Vatican became one of the wealthiest states in the world. The knowledge and personal use of gems was condemned and withheld from the people.

Still, the Italians were very much concerned with the study of gems, and in 1531 Marbodus published a treatise claiming, among other things, that the Diamond had the power to ward off any "nocturnal spectres" (nightmares). It was also, he claimed, the only gem that repulsed Satan both day and night.

Throughout time, the use of gems has persisted. The oldest magic formulas that we can still interpret are from the ancient Sumerian civilization of Babylonia. One of their texts names the Solar Deity as being the one to determine whether a gem would be blessed or cursed.

To the Chinese, Jade was the jewel of heaven. Confucius said, "From all time, sages have compared virtuous humanity with Jade." In the Muhammadan world, there is an orthodox sect called the Pekdah, who from birth to death carry a piece of Jade to enhance their relationship with God. The Persians gave such great credence to Turquoise, for example, that they ranked it along with friendship and the Koran as one of the three most important things necessary to make a good life.

One of the most eminently respected spiritual healers of the Western world in our lifetimes, Dr. Carl Jung, was convinced all myths, fairy tales, and legends actually have roots in truth. His lifetime of study of the human brain, mind, and spirit also convinced him that the mind rules the body.

Emanuel Swedenborg, theological mystic of the 1700s, wrote a twelve-volume work on the actual correspondence of things on Earth with our inner consciousness and with things on other levels of existence. Swedenborg spent the first fifty years of his life engaged in ardent scientific research and then pursued the spiritual quest with the same intelligence and earnestness for the next thirty years.

Some of the fastest-growing churches in America are those that intertwine science and the mystical. The Science of Mind Church, founded by Ernest Holmes, the Rosicrucian Fellowship, founded by Max Heindel, Church of Religious Science, Christian Science, and Unity are all growing. They recognize the positive relationship between the body, mind, and spirit of man to the Universe.

Emerging from the past Age of Taurus (Genesis in the Old Testament, approximately 10,000 B.C.), and the planets' movements through the Age of Pisces that began with the birth of Jesus two thousand years ago, we now come to the New Age of Aquarius. Just as we can look back through our recent history and see why the Dark Ages were really dark, we will be able to see why this New Age is really new.

Everything that man has made on Earth is copied from the patterns of the Universe. We can think or do nothing unless it has first been thought and done by the macrocosm.

Because we still have not really entered the New Age, the esoteric maxim that is the password of understanding among all students of metaphysics, "As above so below," is not fully understood. Since we are very close to the gates of the New Age, we do see and feel its effect long before we arrive. It is this influence we are approaching, the knowledge of which has been passed on to us by every saint, initiate, ascended master, philosopher, poet, guru, or artist since man first spoke. "It is so simple it confounds the wise . . . the Kingdom of Heaven is within YOU."

There is a significant part of the population worldwide who are fearful of straying from their religious tradition. As the lady in the Macon, Georgia, audience asked me, "Do the crystals do the healing, or do the Lawd do the healing?" Even my own son, who is a born-again Christian, is concerned about my healing crystal work. It is not logical to me, however, to separate the crystals from the other minerals and elements that are used in medicine and call them unholy.

The Designing Creative Force (God) has given us the crystals to heal ourselves and invisible energies such as electricity and every other form of healing vibration with which to soothe our souls and heal our bodies.

All "healers," whether we be physicians, counselors, chiropractors, massage therapists, astrologers, nurses, teachers, ministers, palm readers, numerologists, surgeons, or just a loving friend, are only channels for the Cosmic Current.

4/ The Coming of the New Age

"During the last two thousand years, the symbol of the Age of Pisces was the cross. I believe that the crystal will symbolize the next two thousand years, the Age of Aquarius."

—Brett Bravo

▲▲▲

I believe the crystal message is coming through so loud and clear now because the cycles of the heavens have moved. We are moving from one age into another. The Age of Pisces was begun with the birth, or the emergence, of the Christ consciousness, embodied in a human being who preached and taught people about a new way of living. This Age of Pisces had to do with the development of the individual.

Pisces is a constellation in the heavens. The planets moving around us move through these constellations. So for two thousand years, that particular constellation and the way the Earth turned kept the vibration of that constellation focused on Earth. But the Earth is turning in a way and the constellations are moving in cycles to a degree that we will be receiving the vibration of the constellation Aquarius. This turning will also bring two new planets into our solar system, Vulcan and another yet undiscovered. These will bring change to us. We spent the last two thousand years developing the individual person. We have eliminated serfdom and slavery. Monarchy and race consciousness are in their dying throes, and humanity is experiencing personal freedom. The New Age is about the Universal person.

The radio, in which the Quartz crystal frequency transmitted the human voice across invisible space, was the first step toward changing this planet into one world, one race, one people. The telegraph, as a means of communication, was physical, using visible wires. The radio is metaphysical because it uses unseen waves. The radio was a direct result of the planet Uranus, which was first seen in our solar system in 1781, about the time Ben Franklin tied the key to the kite. One hundred years later, Thomas Edison invented the light bulb. We started to feel the influence of the New Age of Aquarius in connection with the advent of the understanding of electricity.

The new planets will also bring changes. In esoteric teaching, there is always a foretelling of the future felt on Earth from one hundred to five hundred years in advance. Occult writings predict that the new ruler of Virgo is in the wings. The name of the unseen planet is Vulcan. It is predicted that great changes will occur with the discovery of this planet. In the coming years, we will feel the distant energy waves from Vulcan as it approaches.

When Pluto entered our galaxy in 1930, it had been preceded by two hundred years of revolution for personal freedom, amid oppression by the monarchy and the church.

The energy wave of Pluto caused transfiguration of the consciousness for several centuries before it was close enough to Earth to be visible.

In planetary language, the description of Pluto's effects on humanity are reorganizing and provoking transition, secret forces of nature and occult sensitivity, regeneration, sexual energy, and transformaton through death and rebirth. In reviewing history over the past fifty years, we can surely see the effects of Pluto's transmission on our world societies.

We have named the places where inner heat, stress, and pressure are expelled from inside the Earth—"volcanos." We have a tendency to judge this action of the Earth to expel fire and hot lava as destructive. We stand in fear and awe of this phenomenon. If we tune in to the metaphoric meanings of Vulcan, it is entirely possible that these random and worldwide eruptions are actually a process of the Earth's inner computer.

For example, in our orbit around our central Sun, the spaceship Earth has a tendency to shift on its axis and to wobble slightly. It may go off course—exactly as some of the satellites that we have launched have done. In order to right itself, it has built-in rockets that blast off. Man has copied this correction process in torpedoes and spacecraft.

If we will constantly keep in mind that everything we invent can be found operating somewhere in nature, we can begin to understand that the patterns of all creation are already a part of the human brain.

The coming of Vulcan into our cycles is preceded by fire. Vulcan is the transforming flame that often accompanies violent explosion. Explosion breaks up old crystallized thought patterns. Fire cleanses and transforms worn-out elements into a totally different form and vibration. Fire and explosion force change. At the beginning, these appear to be negative disasters.

In order to comprehend the nature of Vulcan, observe

the progressive, revitalizing change that has occurred in two explosive areas of human consciousness on Earth. In Europe, consider Germany. In Asia, consider Japan.

Vulcan's effect on our consciousness has been active since early in this century. The German "race consciousness," like that of the Japanese, has been blasted, exploded, and burned into a new and dynamic contribution to the family of man.

Nothing short of an atomic blast could have shaken loose the crystallized vibrations locked into the ethers surrounding those two nations. Vulcan pounded Europe, and especially Germany, on his great anvil to reshape the archetypal patterns. With Japan, it was the transformation of fire, burning away completely not only the archetypal patterns but also the earthly manifestations. The purifying fires of war have released the most magnificent talents and intellect of a brilliant people.

There will continue to be explosions, fires, and restructuring within nations until the old race consciousness is transformed into global consciousness. Vulcan is approaching. This influence will be felt as the time nears for its discovery.

We must accept the frightening fire and explosions that will be necessary to shake us out of our indifferent and indolent slumber. This will occur as a simultaneous evolution on the personal, internal level as well as on global political and galactic levels.

Vulcan, the powerful god of fire, is the guiding planet for the feminine sign of the innocent virgin. Virgo is a negative sign, Vulcan is a positive force. The balance of the combination will free the creative spirit within all Virgo-born.

Dedicated to service, work, and health, the Virgo will find that these three most important necessities for rebuilding in the New Age of Aquarius will be strengthened. Look to all present and future Virgoans as the channels who will accomplish the nitty-gritty details for the transformation and evolution of our bodies, minds, and spirits. Millions of Virgoans worldwide will not be aware of the contracts they have made with themselves and evolution, but the few who do will surrender themselves to the task.

The gem that is receiving and conducting the transmissions from Vulcan is a tricolor stone of rather recent acceptance, the Tourmaline. It is a unique crystal of the hexagonal (trigonal) family.

This gem has been known since antiquity in the Mediterranean region and was imported from Sri Lanka by the Dutch around 1700. Its rarity has been recently diminished by vast discoveries in South Africa, Brazil, and the United States.

It is in Southern California that the gem is being introduced to society at large. This magnificent vacation area is the natural home of the beautiful Tourmaline. In the small town of Fallbrook, which lies between Los Angeles and San Diego, there is a family-owned mine and retail display of Tourmaline jewelry made from the nearby Pala mines.

The triple colors, often found in one Tourmaline crystal, are bringing the body, mind, and spirit messages to many souls worldwide. Many of the top names in scientific research have come to the West Coast, of California. Nowhere on Earth have there been drawn together so many "strangers" who "know" each other. The holistic health movement can be traced to doctors, dentists, scholars, chiropractors, and nurses from all over the world who have come to Tourmaline country.

The foremost practitioners of Humanist Psychology, Carl Rogers, Everell Shostrom, and others, have all found Southern California to be the right "climate" to holistically explore the human mind, heart, and spirit.

The approach of Vulcan, the planetary ruler of Vir-

▲▲▲

goans, will bring into action the true lessons and challenges that Virgos everywhere have chosen. That is, to be in service, working towards the health of society and of the planet Earth. The trigonal vibration of Tourmaline will conduct and amplify the Vulcan message.

Part Two

UNLOCKING THE CRYSTAL SECRETS

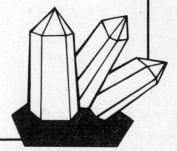

5/ Choosing Your Crystal

"Is it not of timely interest to inquire—having the results of modern investigations into radioactivity and force rays—whether precious stones may not be capable of exerting therapeutic influences?"

—William T. Fernie, MD

▲▲▲

Everyone has designed and created their own bodies. You know every cell in your body on a subconscious or superconscious level. No one knows your body as well as you do. To say to anyone outside yourself, "Make me well," is to deny your own power of healing.

Mother Earth has provided us with every tool we could possibly need to build a healthy body. The plant and mineral kingdoms offer every medicine that is prescribed.

Crystals contain chemical elements that will trigger within

us a resonant response when stimulated by the planetary rays. As with any tool, the crystal must be used. Like the hammer and nail, cooperation must exist between the tool and the builder.

The simple first step in your crystal education will be to find just the right stone for you, which I can guarantee will be an interesting quest. Maybe the stone you seek will be linked to something from your past, a special gem you may have had when you were a child, or perhaps it is one you have always liked.

Don't be afraid to make your own choice. I really believe that people are extremely wise and intuitive. Most of us don't live our lives that way, however. We don't do what we like, because our early training has taught us a lot of rules about what's good and what's bad. We are fearful about indulging ourselves. If you like it, it's probably bad. Actually, it's not that way at all. If we just follow our natural instincts, we will make good choices because we are naturally good. After all, we are replicas of the Designing Creative Force of the Universe.

One of the drawbacks that I've found in working with people who are not accustomed to metaphysics or spirituality is they have a tendency to be a little superstitious. They often say, "Oh, well, I was born in February, so my stone is an Amethyst." I want to remind people over and over again, only pick a stone if it turns you on. When it comes to choosing a crystal, nothing is more important than liking it. You should be able to say, "I feel good with this one, I like it, it's the one I want." If it's not the best one for you, there are many other major stones described in Part III you may look at before making your decision.

Everybody understands their so-called birth stones. They were the gems assigned to the month you were born that are ruled by a certain planet. We've talked about birth stones and Sun signs all our lives. But birth stones are not relevant anymore because the jewelers have changed the months that the stones go with for whatever was convenient for them and whatever the vagaries of supply and demand were at the time. I found twelve official birthstone lists throughout a 5000-year history, where birth stones changed from country to country, and from translation to translation.

The long and short of it is, don't limit yourself in your choice of a stone by what you have been led to believe is the right one for you. There is a message in every jewel. There is a certain stone for every vibration, with a correlation between the vibration of the planets, the gems, and you.

The best place to begin searching for your first gem is a lapidary shop. Most people don't know exactly what a crystal is. Jewelry stores usually sell only faceted stones, so if you want to start by looking in a jewelry store at some of the finest cut stones, you can begin to get an idea of which ones appeal to you the most. But these polished, cut, and faceted gems can be very expensive and there is no need to begin your gem education by spending a lot of money. In a lapidary shop you can buy a small piece of the raw, uncut gem to which you have felt an attraction. These rough crystals are every bit as powerful as the cut gems. You can experiment with them without having to make a large financial commitment.

Almost every little town has a rock shop or a gem and mineral society. Museums often have a gemological display in which you can find out which gem really turns you on. You can even get good color photographs in books at the library that can help you decide. Simply by looking at the pictures in a book you can actually receive the vibration as it has been caught by the camera.

After you've done some investigating, call around to the different places that have crystals for sale and ask them if they have an Amethyst crystal, for instance, or do they have an Emerald crystal. Ask for something in the natural form, which will be less expensive than the faceted gem.

Let's say now you have picked the crystal that your intuitive, natural knowing has told you is the right one. What next? You will begin to know this special gem and the secrets locked inside it that are only waiting for your use. Don't worry about whether you know enough to begin your gem education. The lessons of the gems come through in spite of ourselves. Specific meditations for each crystal are found in Part III.

Before you turn to Part III and the healing crystal meditations, here are some important instructons on how to treat your new crystal.

Before you begin using your new crystal, it should be cleansed. Your crystal was touched by many people before you found it and brought it home. It was mined by one person, handled by two or three people at the time, then cut and faceted by still another. It was packed and shipped by someone, unpacked by others, and transported wherever you finally found it. It was also priced and laid out on the shelf. Heaven knows how many people handled it before you bought it.

When people buy my healing crystal jewelry, they always want to put it right on their bodies. And I say, okay, that's all right, I don't blame you for that because you're excited to have it. But when you get home tonight, do this: Clean this crystal. Don't keep it around indefinitely without taking care of that.

There is no one set way to deprogram or cleanse a crystal, whether it's a colored crystal or a Clear Quartz. But there are certain easy methods that I have used that I will explain, and you can choose the way you like. I always wash my crystals in salt water and place them outside to absorb the ultraviolet rays that are there day or night. Because I live close to the beach, ocean water is easy for me to get, but table salt added to water will do just as well. Lay your crystal out all night. Whether it is cloudy or not, the ultraviolet rays will still be there, emitted by the Moon at night and by the Sun during the day.

The crystals are basically born in water. Cleansing the crystals in salt water returns them to their embryonic fluid. When I take a bath, it's the same thing. I'm washing my aura and going back to my embryonic state, which is pure simplicity and pure spirit.

But you may have other feelings and other memories. The Indians burned sage and held the crystal in the smoke. Some people prefer placing their crystal in running water or a clear mountain stream. There are even new, modern high-tech ways to deprogram and cleanse crystals, such as with an electromagnetic VCR head cleaner. I use the method of salt water, Sun, and Moon for twenty-four hours because I am a person who is into cycles. I relate to the movement of the Earth and stars and the plan of the overall galaxy. I like ritual. It makes me feel good, as if I am in some kind of cycle.

You may want to bury your crystal back into the Earth. Even a pot of soil will isolate the gem and rejuvenate it with Nature's own vibrations. An abalone shell can be used as a container for cedar chips, which can be purchased at your local nursery, and burned for their purifying smoke. However you decide to cleanse your crystal, do it as a personal ceremony in which you and the crystal act together. Remember, this is a lifetime healing partnership. Consider this a marriage, with the same kind of commitment. Keep your crystal with you all the time, sleep with it, bathe with it, and enjoy it.

When you have chosen your crystal, you may want to know exactly what it means, immediately. You do know already on a superconscious level what you need. If you look in Part III to find the meaning and discover that on a conscious level you don't understand the connection, be patient with yourself. Trust your higher knowing and trust the crystal because I may not have described your need in words you expected to hear. Do not reject your knowing because the so-called experts, including myself, do not have all the answers, yet. You may be able to add your experience to our data.

For instance, if you chose Emerald, which will encourage you to "come clean with the truth" and to give out love, and you think you already do that, you may have a tendency to reject your choice. The Emerald also has an effect on the bones and spine. There may be a stressful situation occurring in your life that is directly related to backache and misalignment of the skeletal system that directly relates on a subconscious level to your misunderstanding of a situation. Your body is responding with aches and pains to the fact that you have not examined everything and come completely clean with the truth about it. You also may be feeling you are not getting enough love, which makes you unwilling to give out love.

There are levels of understanding that the crystal will help you to as you do the daily meditations.

Are you drawn to more than one stone? My clients often ask if they can choose two. My procedure is to recommend making a choice between them and doing only one healing before beginning the second. The superconscious mind can make a decision on what is most important. It is only the conscious mind that gets confused.

Focusing the energy one step at a time is the most successful. When you feel ready, proceed to the next crystal. Some needs will change. I personally always feel a need for the Amethyst. But I do at other times use Pink Tourmaline and Kunzite as my intuition dictates. I used Pink Tourmaline for over two years, even though I continued wearing the Amethyst. After you are experienced with the crystals, you will be able to diagnose for yourself which one you need at any given time.

I have not experienced any negative results from using more than one stone at a time. However, I do not mix different vibrations in my healing crystal jewelry. To the beginner, I would recommend using only one crystal at a time.

If you have picked a colored crystal, you have chosen one that carries its own vibration and is transmitting certain rays from the planet with which it is cosmically connected. For instance, the Ruby transmits the red ray from Mars. Now somebody's going to ask, "How do you know that a Ruby is transmitting that vibration? How do you know that the red ray comes from the planet Mars?" And I have to say, not only is it ancient knowledge, but every astronomer calls Mars the red planet. They're not astrologers, they are scientists.

Ancient manuscripts show that certain crystals are transmitting correlating rays from the planets. Just because they're ancient manuscripts does not mean they were primitive societies. The Atlanteans probably knew exactly how to direct energy through a Ruby crystal much the same as we know laser surgery today.

Now, when it comes to a colored crystal, they also pick up other energies, but what they are programmed for is what they will do. So, you can't just put a program into a colored crystal, because it's already programmed to affect certain parts of your body. That's the difference between the Clear Quartz and the colored crystal.

Clear Quartz is like aspirin or a good cup of tea. It relieves the symptoms. Now there are a lot of people that are studying quartz who are saying it will do absolutely everything. But if that were true, we wouldn't have colored crystals.

If you are using a colored crystal, I have written some very simple sentences to go with each crystal that is included in this book. These sentences are used with a seven-minute meditation that I developed by combining years of research with my experience working with hundreds of clients and their response to the healing colored crystals.

When I say meditation, a lot of people immediately will think of transcendental meditation, where you blank out the mind completely and forget where you are, who you are, and what's going on. They think it is hard and they don't want to try it. When I say meditation, what I mean is to simply contemplate the crystal, which is the first step in developing a relationship with it. At least give yourself a chance to respond to the crystal by using the meditation that is suggested in Part III. If this doesn't feel comfortable after twenty-eight days, design your own meditation.

After you have found your crystal, brought it home with you, and cleansed it, you have begun what you will soon find to be an enduring relationship with it. Hold it in your hand and look at it. Each of my meditations with the crystals begins with looking inside it, synchronizing your vibration with the gem. Something happens as you gaze into your gem. You will find yourself lost in the crystal. You will feel something come over you. It is wonderment as you get in tune with Earth and wind and fire.

The sentences that I have written for the purpose of contemplation with each crystal arose from the positive aspects that I have discovered through my own contemplation with them. After you have gazed into your crystal for at least one full minute, your electromagnetic field will change its vibration as the crystal vibration begins to modify it.

The Quartz crystal is used as a master stone as it transmits a general amount of all the cosmic rays. In this state the crystal may be programmed by your thought power to focus and direct energy toward your specific requirements or needs.

The crystalline structure of colored stones denotes a preprogrammed quality. This means that their geometric lattice is crystallized in such a way as to refract and transmit the energy of a specific color ray. Each planet and certain areas of the Cosmos are directing energy rays toward each other and toward Earth that have an effect on our Mental, Spiritual, Emotional, and Physical Bodies. A few of these that scientists know about are ultraviolet, infrared, gamma and X rays, radio waves, alpha, beta, and so forth.

The colored crystals transmit and direct these rays. From close contact with these gems the body intuitively begins to harmonize on the same frequency.

6/ Twenty-Eight Days to a Miracle: Seven-Minute Healing Meditations

"We are called upon to exert effort in working with the positive vibrations of the gems, with knowledge, visualization, concentration, and desire for good."

—Brett Bravo

▲▲▲

Before you begin your meditations, you will already have chosen the gem that corresponds to your personal vibration, following the guidance of your superconscious. Remember that the crystal can be in any form, rough or faceted, mounted or natural. There is no need for you to go out and purchase an expensive cut gem in a gold setting.

It is best to do this meditation ritual in complete privacy. Each of the meditations begins with gazing into the crystal for at least one full minute, which synchronizes the gem's vibration to your own and produces an "alpha" wave of receptivity. After one week you will have established a response pattern. Upon sitting down thereafter, your subconscious will be attentive.

Don't limit your time gazing into the crystal to only one minute if you feel you are comfortable with more time. You could sit for an hour and it would help you immensely. I shorten the time to only one minute especially for busy people who always say they don't have time to meditate. After synchronizing with your crystal, lie down on the floor. I suggest this position because most people don't ever lie on the floor. The subconscious mind takes this as a cue that you mean business. And lying on the floor makes it too hard to go to sleep.

Place the crystal between your lower ribs and your navel (the area of the solar plexus). Cover the gem with your palm and repeat aloud the sentence that goes with your specific crystal (found in Part III). Do this seven times, or for two minutes.

There are valid reasons for decreeing aloud the vibrational message within a gem. When we speak, our words carry vibrations that travel through the ethers of the air about the Earth and into the Cosmos. This is a scientifically measurable fact.

The creation of all that we know came about in the beginning by the spoken word of the Mother-Father Creators, as was written in all the ancient spiritual writings, East and West. First came the DESIRE to create and then came the WORD. The vibrations of the words caused sound waves, which are patterns of energy. The energy produced matter.

All spiritual groups throughout history have used words spoken as mantras, responsive readings, chants, or songs to reach the Original Creator. If one word causes a small vibration, when that word is repeated, the vibration is also repeated. It is multiplied if it bounces into the vibrations of the word spoken before it. When the vibration is multiplied and the energy increased, more matter is produced.

As the vibrations continue to ripple out and multiply, they geometrically square each other. There will occur a gradual but visible change in the molecular structure of the body and brain that is within range of the vibration. Of course, this is also true of any negative words. They create negative results and molecular changes that are destructive.

The cosmic rays that are invisible will penetrate the crystal, which becomes a transmitter for those rays. They will go right into the fuse box of your Emotional Body when you hold the crystal against the solar plexus. This ensures all the breakers are working so that the cosmic rays will affect the physical body. It is important, for this reason, to begin the meditation exercises with the solar plexus.

Hold the crystal over your heart and recite the specific affirmation for another two minutes.

Hold the crystal against your forehead, the area of the pineal gland that is called the third eye. Repeat the final affirmation.

As soon as the third affirmation is finished, write your thoughts in a notebook. Don't try to monitor or judge these thoughts. Don't try to analyze them. In time they will assume a pattern and you will begin to recognize the information that is coming to you just as in your dreams.

Keep the gem with you at all times. It doesn't have to be worn as a piece of jewelry. You can keep it in your pocket, wallet, or purse, or pin it to your clothing next to the skin. Sleep with it under your pillow.

Within a week a breakthrough can occur. After twenty-one days, extreme changes can take place. This twenty-eight-day program has been beneficial to many of my clients, who have said, "I can't tell you what that did for my life."

They just spent seven minutes a day for twenty-eight days in direct communication with the Cosmos.

Each gem has its positive effect on our total being. Because of the interior angles of molecule construction, the vibration of certain gems will not benefit us as much as the exact gem would. In certain instances, the vibrational frequency is too high, and we feel a tension, as we automatically strive to raise our own to its level. This is not negative, but unnecessary. We have only to listen to our own communication centers to realize if the stress is more advanced than we can accommodate comfortably. A certain amount of stress is absolutely imperative to growth.

These things do not automatically occur, without effort. The user of a gem must consciously cooperate with the transmitter. If your receiving station is unwittingly shut down, no messages can be transmitted efficiently. Fortunately the cosmic rays penetrate to some degree even the most unconscious. In metaphysical terms, compare receiving a telepathic feeling that someone is in your thoughts versus receiving an actual call on the telephone from the person. The physical, conscious acknowledgment of each crystal's healing properties makes its transmission more effective.

When the formula for meditation I have devised is used regularly in connection with a corresponding time of quiet, amazing changes occur in the life and health pattern. The personal vibration of the life spirit will be raised to a higher octave. At this point, the personal vibration has more power and can travel farther. Things at great distance can be affected. Telepathic messages can be sent directly and with purpose. There is an entry point in space that can be reached to connect our own vibrational intelligence to the Universal Consciousness. This entry point can only be reached through conscious effort on our part.

I had a client, a woman in her late sixties, who never

claimed interest in metaphysics. She reported to me a chronically inflamed esophagus and an enlarged opening into the stomach that was very painful when she ate or drank.

She was being treated by a physician who administered rather large doses of tranquilizers, which were beginning to inhibit her work as a creative clothing designer. She had been treated medically for more than six months with no improvement.

I suggested an Aquamarine crystal for her to wear at the thymus (throat chakra). She was a very mild-mannered and retiring person on the outside, but underneath, the caldron was boiling. She had become increasingly worried over a lawsuit, the pending outcome of which was creating excessive concern.

The Aquamarine transmits on the blue-violet ray from the planet Venus. It works on the pineal gland located in the forebrain (known in Eastern philosophy as the "third eye") to bring relief from anxiety and peace of mind.

She wore the crystal constantly, faithfully performing the meditation cycle I suggested. At the end of the month, her checkup with her doctor showed vast improvement and she stopped all further medication.

Another client of mine was a gentleman in his late sixties who was troubled with a twenty-year history of respiratory problems, including severe bronchial infections. He had been treated by numerous physicians with medications and strict diets, but the coughing, wheezing, and labored breathing persisted.

Eventually, he was ordered to move to the dry, inland climate of California and to retire from his stressful oc-cupation. But even after five years of sunshine and quiet living, his condition was only slightly improved.

At first he didn't even want to have a psychic reading because he said he didn't believe in the process. I suggested that he at least keep an Amethyst crystal in his shirt pocket and sleep with it under his pillow, and not to be without it. He didn't do the meditation, "forgot" to keep the crystal with him, and after one month his condition wasn't very much better.

The Amethyst transmits the violet ray from the planet Mercury. It not only works to clarify communication, it is also a protector of the respiratory system.

I convinced him to wear the crystal on a chain around his neck. He left grumbling, "This is ridiculous," but agreed to think about the possibility of the transmission of cosmic rays.

I didn't hear from him for several months, but finally received a call from his wife, who called to report that at his six-month checkup, the doctor had been quite surprised at his improved physical condition.

The old gentleman had always been judgmental and self-righteous. His family each told me individually of a great softening in his overall attitude after wearing the crystal.

Another case history is that of a young man, thirty-five years old, with a lifetime of allergies. He wanted a psychic reading that would suggest a gem-crystal for him, but I felt he could intuitively choose the right one for himself.

After inspecting each of my twenty-eight crystals, he ultimately chose a blue Tourmaline. He agreed to do the seven-minute daily meditation and to keep a notebook of any thoughts that might come into his mind afterward.

The reading I did for him brought to light a great sadness dating back to his childhood. When he fastened the crystal around his neck, he subconsciously put it into his mouth.

After one month of using the Tourmaline in meditation and taking notes, he reported total cessation of his allergies, even though it was high-pollen season.

The young man found that his allergies were actually

the only acceptable way he allowed himself to cry. When he put the Tourmaline into his mouth, it triggered child-hood memories that brought a flood of tears.

The blue Tourmaline, transmitting a multi-ray from the yet undiscovered planet named Vulcan, balances the phys-ical body with three invisible bodies, working especially on the release of tears.

The Emerald became an especially powerful crystal for me personally at a time when I had to rethink some im-portant decisions.

The Emerald transmits a green ray from Saturn, the planet identified by astrologers as the "strict teacher." The vibration of the Emerald insists that the wearer "Come clean with the truth." Physically speaking, it affects the skeleton, bones, spine, teeth, and knees.

I had a problem with the structure of my knees disin-tegrating. Not only did my painful condition prohibit me from playing tennis, which I loved, but doctors told me unless I had an operation, I would be an invalid.

After the second month of using the meditation and wearing the crystal at the heart level, I noticed a great improvement in my knees. My friends also commented on how much more loving I had become. The Emerald forced me to become more honest with myself.

I have done hundreds of readings for people I have never even met and many more face-to-face. I have en-couraged feedback on the accuracy and the usefulness of these readings. The most dramatic testimonies often come from men. It is astonishing how the male polarity can do an absolute about-face when something is presented in a clear way. The left-brain, logic-oriented male makes sig-nificant and steadfast decisions when the right-brain agrees. This appears to work in reverse with women, with similar results.

One of my executive clients reported to me the results of his twenty-eight-day meditation with the Blue Topaz.

He had chosen this crystal by intuition and from really liking the color. (It is sky blue and very clear.) It is no coincidence that it has an effect of calming the nervous system, positive self-improvement, and determined awake consciousness.

I had suggested that he do the meditation exercise first thing every morning. All of his writings each day included a comprehensive list of things he intended to accomplish for the day. After I listened patiently to thirty days of this, I felt the exercise had totally failed to calm him, nor had it distracted his left brain. It had served as a time to focus on "business as usual." Of course in the long run, organization does have a calming effect.

I suggested that if he was willing, we could try the exercise at night before bed, in the usual manner, holding the Blue Topaz on the solar plexus, heart, and forehead.

He agreed, and within a week he was reporting unusual dreams. They were very vivid in his mind upon awakening and were very helpful to him.

Many of his previous notes after the exercise were about other people. I suggested this exercise was for getting in touch with HIMSELF. The nervous or high-action person often takes no time for this. The next notes were all to begin with "I . . ."

This proved so successful I learned a completely new approach for helping the crystal work with the invisible Mental Body. The most miraculous part of this example is that this man was affected by the first month of using this Blue Topaz on a very subliminal level.

The second month he was beginning to read quietly, watching less and less TV. He began to appreciate quiet. His notes after each seven-minute exercise began to start with his first name, and he was writing in a most unusual way: waiting for each word as though it were dictated. He was getting in touch with his higher mind at last. He reports a feeling of calmness prevails.

Now I ask my clients to use the crystal morning or evening for seven minutes and choose the time that feels best. I also suggest that they begin all their note writing after each exercise with "I . . ."

Often the results people experience after meditation are not what they expected at all. Many of my clients report to me extraordinary dreams, heightened sensations of color, feelings of peace and connectedness, and actual visions.

Susan meditated twice a day with the Amethyst her husband had bought her. A very visual person, she saw pictures in which the souls of people formed a circle around the Earth. They spoke to her and she felt she knew them, which made her feel very comforted.

She also noticed that the Amethyst's message of enhanced communication affected other members of her family just by its presence. Her teenage son began writing poetry.

Donna chose a pink Tourmaline that she kept with her at all times, tucking it into her bra where it could be held close to the heart chakra. She slept with it, did the prescribed meditation, and was hardly ever without it. She experienced a radical release from anger almost immediately. Pent-up emotions poured from her as she freed herself from long-held but unrecognized resentments. She realized through working with the Tourmaline that she had been burying her emotions, pretending they didn't matter. Able to identify her sadness as coming from "losing the dream," she brought her anger to the surface at last. The process of release had just begun for her, but constantly repressed emotion would have harmed her physically before long.

Clients and friends of mine from all over the world and all walks of life share the crystal information I have given them with others.

A friend of mine told me of a chance meeting with a past acquaintance whom she had not seen for eleven years.

She explained that she had ordered a Kunzite crystal from a metaphysical conference held by the Colorado School of Mines in Golden, Colorado. As she was picking up the package containing the specimen at the post office, the old friend, who was an alcoholic, happened in. They talked, and he told her his problem drinking had caused him so much turmoil that he really wished to stop. She unwrapped her package, gave him the crystal, and asked him to keep it on him as an aid in attaining soberness. Three months later his wife called, reporting that he had been dry ever since the day he received the Kunzite.

Of course, crystals are very much a part of my daily personal rituals. I wear the Amethyst and meditate with it because I realize that in order to be a good healer, I have to get my judgmental nature out of the conversation when I'm dealing with a client. I have to allow myself to get into their body, to get into their subconscious mind, to get into their heart and feel how it feels. I couldn't do that if I didn't think purely and get rid of my judgmental nature. I also wear a pink Tourmaline crystal on a long chain so that it's right at my heart level. I'm working on the understanding of the Emotional Body, in connection with the Spirit Body. The pink Tourmaline, I believe, is transmitting rays from an area in the Universe and from a specific planet that we have not yet seen, Vulcan.

Scientists know there's another planet, and I believe from my experience with this crystal and from my clients' experiences with this crystal that the planet is already sending cosmic rays to Earth and that Tourmaline is transmitting these cosmic rays. You know, in the series *Star Trek*, Mr. Spock was supposedly from Vulcan. He was very logical, analytical, and unemotional so he could figure things out without getting emotionally involved.

Vulcan is transmitting an energy to balance the body, and it does this by transformation of fire. When I talk to my clients about "going through the fire," they may think that's terrible. But I'm talking about the fire of transformation. I want desperately to balance that Emotional Body of mine, because as soon as that gets more balanced, I'll be able to move forward in my own evolution and be able to be more centered so that I can do better work. I won't be as susceptible to the negative energy that I can create with my Emotional Body, which I've found to be so destructive. I wear the pink Tourmaline, and by looking at it, thinking of it, knowing it's there, holding it against my heart, picking it up and holding it in my hand, I'm constantly reminded that I am studying myself.

I have crystals all over my house, wherever I am, whether I'm in the bathroom, in my living room, in my bedroom, or in the kitchen. I look at the crystals, and because I've studied them so long, I know what they're telling me. I just receive their message in a constant affirmation. I get uplifted from their visual beauty. Just looking at them is like looking at a beautiful flower or clouds in the sky; they have everything in them.

All aspects of daily life can be beneficially affected through awareness of the secrets of the crystals. In the day-to-day business world, for instance, let's say there's an important meeting coming up. You really want to express yourself clearly and succinctly, so you could take an Amethyst with you and ask for its communicating vibration to assist you. Take a seven-minute break in the morning before the day begins, work with this crystal, then keep it near you, if possible at the throat chakra. Expect what you say at the meeting to be coming from the pure essence of your spirit, and there is no doubt that your presentation will be the very best you've ever given.

A lot of psychologists and other "brain people" would say that's just positive thinking. You could take a penny or any rock off the beach and it would have the same effect. I don't think so. Each particular crystal means something to the psyche of the person using it. It's a method of focusing certain energies that are invisible. You are acting on a level of faith and surrender, asking and expecting to receive.

The other examples that come to mind are rather convincing. They concern areas where positive thinking could not have been a factor.

This is a testimonial sent to me from Santa Fe, New Mexico—

"Rosita, the Pediatric Nurse's Aide":

Some time ago I was given a one-inch-diameter Rose Quartz crystal ball. As I carried it in the pocket of my uniform, it became very special to me. I was told that it transmitted the pink ray that brought a gentleness into the way I could love myself and others. Because it was small, I gave it the Spanish diminutive name "Rosita."

In the pediatric intensive care unit, tiny premature infants stay with us in their isolettes. It is in these small plastic boxes, with controlled humidity, oxygen content, and temperature, that the babies make their home for weeks until they are strong enough to go home.

An infant is constantly monitored with state-of-the-art technology for electrocardiac impulses, internal temperature, etc. Nurses and doctors know the adverse effects external stimulation has on these delicate little beings. Bumping the isolette, touching their skin, or loud noises will startle them enough to alter their vital signs to an alarming degree.

While caring for these infants, I've been led to warm "Rosita" in my hand and then place it in the hand of an irritable baby. It fits into the palm of a two-and-one-half-pound "preemie."

The immediate results were impressive to me:

heart rates stabilized, respirations became even and unlabored, which decreased oxygen consumption and allowed them to be weaned from the air sooner. Their level of irritability and excitability decreased, which led to an increase in feeding tolerance. This helps them to gain weight. In every instance there seemed to be a calming, relaxing effect.

My experiment with the babies is ongoing and I consider it one of the most exciting aides I have had in twelve years of nursing.

—**Cheri Davenport**
Sr. Pediatric Nurse

At this point I want you to become excited, knowing that others have experienced the gentle persuasion and healing energies of the crystal secrets.

Often these adventures into the Cosmic Connection we make with our Earth and our Universe are transforming and dramatic.

You knew you were ready to invest in yourself when you chose to read this book.

7/ Understanding the Yin-Yang Principle: Enhancing Sexuality with the Love Crystals

"Good sex means better health."

—Eric Berne, MD

▲▲▲

The balancing of the yin-yang or the male-female polarity within each of us is the primary function of evolution. It is also the answer to the perfection of the human physical creation.

The involution into matter by the once androgynous "spirit" had to be experienced through many lifetimes as either male or female. In this way, each facet of the Divine

Mother-Father Creator could be experienced by we children. The force and will to action of the masculine coupled with the creative, receptive intuition of the feminine is the simple formula of the "secret forces of nature."

Women have been very busy developing the "inner man" in order to take on added responsibility in world evolution. Technology has made it possible for her to be relieved of certain home and family-oriented, mundane tasks so she may develop her potential as a cocreator of the future rather than through procreation only.

Observing the developed countries on Earth, we see that women have made great strides in becoming workers and builders in their homes, marriages, careers, and communities. As women shoulder their responsibility for masculine evolution, it automatically follows that men will have to learn to nurture themselves much as women have always done for each other.

What appeared to be the breakdown of the nuclear family is the next step in balancing the male and female within us. The female has been in a subservient role for several thousand years. We know that there have been past times when the females were the rulers and everything was matriarchal. But in order to balance the male energy and to give males a chance to develop themselves in their assertiveness and creativeness, the female took the lesser role.

A lot of women have been very angry about this, so they had a revolution. Well, that's all in Divine order, because it was time for that revolution. The female emerging again into positions of power has taken back more of the masculine energy, forcing the males into nurturing themselves, something they weren't able to do while they were developing their masculine energy.

Adornment and the wearing of crystals and precious metals give generous clues to understanding the evolution of the species as well as the progress of the male and female.

Imagine Neanderthal women or men stringing the first pieces of bone, wood, and seeds together. What was their inspiration? Was their primitive instinct developed enough to know that they were channeling the vibrations of the nature spirits, whose job it is to inhabit and direct all nature?

Stones and rocks began to appear in early man's jewelry. The discovery of metals created a quantum leap in both evolution and adornment. The exciting thing to me is not the progress of humanity in learning to make things, but the opposite. I believe that by keeping these spirits and vibrations close to their bodies, the ornaments themselves increased early man's ability to learn.

The introduction of gold, silver, bronze (copper and tin), and brass (copper and zinc) to body ornament paralleled a definite increase in the technical intellect of our ancestors. Most historians will claim that brain development preceded the smelting of ore. I believe that the vibrations received from the metal increased the knowledge of the wearer through its own molecules.

Inert material? No. Nothing is without life and everything is vibration. Gold grows in the Earth in crystal form inside of which is an unchanging measurement of geometry vibrating at a constant rate. Gold speaks to our intellect through our skin sensors. It is the same with every metal and every crystal.

Precious gems and metals are not only precious because of their price. They are expensive because they are desirable. They are desirable because they have messages within their vibrations, like a code. The more intellectually evolved humans are, the more evolved their crystals will be. The great spiritual Law of Attraction is that we attract what we are.

The places of adornment on the body have changed a great deal in the last two hundred years, corresponding to the shift in consciousness necessary for the Aquarian Age.

The great rulers of ancient history, including those of primitive tribes, originally used the head as a place of adornment. We can trace this habit from prehistoric crowns of animal heads to carved wooden and straw crowns in Africa, the golden headdresses of the pharaohs of Egypt, and even the jeweled crown of the present-day Queen of England.

Today, men and women have three basic areas of the body that are instinctively adorned with gold, silver, and gems. The throat, which in occult knowledge is the "power center" of communication, is the most favored, as it has been for at least five thousand years. As a result, communication has reached to outer space.

A recent resurgence in the popularity of gold chains has made it common to see men wearing throat and neck adornment in our Western society. Since gold is a masculine metal and women are wearing the same chains, we can see that both men and women are understanding the true masculine principle.

What makes gold a masculine metal? In occult-wisdom writings, the color of the metal corresponds to the Sun, which is the vital, masculine yang force. The color of silver corresponds to the nurturing and intuitive, emotional Moon, which is the spiritual, feminine yin force.

The second area of adornment most popular today is over the heart. Men wear lapel pins over the heart area to indicate membership in clubs. Women wear brooches, pins, and long necklaces. Men carry silver or gold writing pens in the breast pocket. Gold pocket watches were very stylish for years.

The third area where jewelry is often worn today is the left wrist. In esoteric knowledge of this area, the receiving hand is the left hand and the giving hand is the right hand. By wearing gold, silver, and gems on the left wrist, the vibrational messages are carried through the pulse artery, directly to the heart.

Traditionally, the wedding ring has been worn on the left, receiving hand. The wrist watch has always been worn on the left pulse point of all right-handed persons. Early watches included seventeen-jewel movement for best time-keeping, while today's watches use Quartz. Because the masculine, active energy has been imperative to stimulate rapid advancements, the metal most often used is gold. The gold vibration moves forward aggressively, with energy and will.

The skin has eyes, ears, and other sensory perceptions; the blind can attest to this. They must develop and rely on their nonvisual senses. The vibration of certain metallic crystals (all gems contain metallic mineral substances of some kind) against or near the skin actually makes a difference in the chemical balance of the brain and the body.

The ability of the "common people" to wear precious metal and gems has revolutionized the Western world. By shifting the emphasis from head to throat to heart and receiving hand, we are opening up the areas of skin sensors to receive the new message of the Age of Aquarius. That message is cooperation, agreement, and partnership among nations, planets, galaxies, and lovers.

The New Age is the age of universal citizens. I don't consider myself an American only. I consider myself a global resident. I expect to be traveling in space and saying, "I'm from the Earth; are you from Venus?"

There are two unusual glands in the human body that offer clues to the effect of the crystal vibration on the mind. They are small duplicates of the male and female genitalia. These glands are the masculine pineal, located almost exactly in the center of the head between the base of the skull and the nasal opening, and the feminine pituitary, closer to the front of the skull.

The Western mystic, Max Heindel, founder of the Rosicrucian Fellowship, stated that the pineal is ruled by the planet Neptune. Its secretions affect the physical and mental development of cells in the reproductive organs. He maintains that when the pineal is more highly developed in an individual, it increases in size, enabling the person to become clairvoyant, telepathic, intuitive, and spiritually inspired. It is found to be small or lacking in the mentally retarded.

The Neptunian pineal crystal is being activated now in the male brain to produce intuitive, emotional, creative, nonlogical thought. Since Neptune moved into our solar system in 1846, vibrations have been felt in the crystals of the pineal gland. The technology produced by men to relieve women of time-consuming drudgery is a perfect indication of the marvelous and balanced way the switch in consciousness is taking place within the male mind. The imaginative, creative, social, and intuitive powers of the pineal vibration are being stimulated.

There is an apparent dichotomy in that the masculine gland controls all the properties attributed to the feminine mind as described by research today. Analysts, philosophers, and esoteric writers agree that each man must develop the feminine part within himself to be truly well-balanced.

The pituitary gland has been well-studied and is found to be the distributor of chemicals taken from food, as well as the hormones regulating muscle, tissue, and bone growth. Dwarfism is caused by an undeveloped pituitary. This gland resembles the female sex organ. According to occult writers, it is ruled by the planet Uranus.

In studying both the pituitary and pineal glands, it is interesting to note that there are actual crystals formed within them that are visible upon dissection. The pituitary crystals have been receiving active vibrations of Uranus since we first noticed that planet's entry into our galaxy in 1781. For at least two hundred years, the crystals of the pituitary gland have been receiving the vibrations of Uranus, resulting in a complete change on the Earth and in the lives of women.

Esoteric philosophers say that when the brain evolves to the point that the pineal and pituitary glands unite, as male and female unite sexually, we will approach androgyny, that basic state from which we came.

In the meantime, love, passion, and proper channeling of the creative/sexual Kundalini energy is still a challenge to the human race.

The giving we do in a state of passion offers total surrender of the self, much as Christ gave on the cross. The misunderstanding and misuse of the sexual creative power is the most mysterious to us. We can only experience the fulfillment of unity when we totally surrender our will to control another.

The death of selfish or purely material desire must occur within all of us, to be reborn as a spiritual desire for creative, caring love.

Conventional fears and inhibitions, self-consciousness, or judgment are lost in our passion. What we gain, whether in sexual or other creative expressions, is that elated, pure, and creative state-of-being known as self-satisfaction, not to be confused with the counterfeit emotion of conceit.

The element of fire in our lives produces a physical and emotional heat. It also produces light. The fire element is necessary in the everyday life of each individual as it manifests the will to live vibrating from the red ray of the planet Mars and the burgundy ray of Pluto.

The red ray is a primary color. It creates a primal instinctual response in each of us to survive and to recreate ourselves so that our vibration remains active in the Universe through our children and future generations.

This red ray of fire also ignites a flame of passion that must be in a state of explosion for the burst of energy that creates either a new physical being on Earth or a new vision, thought, or action. The energy of the red ray affirms new life. The season of spring begins with Aries, ruled by the planet Mars, a time bursting forth with blossoms and leaves. Impregnation of the blossoms is done by the bees as their response to the Mars energy. "Busy as a bee" is an apt description of the positive red ray Mars energy. All of the plant and animal kingdoms respond to the vibrations of Mars during this cycle of recreating themselves.

The burgundy vibration of Pluto is in operation with Mars for many months when the human reproductive cycle begins. The burgundy ray is the deep dark red of sexual surrender. It is the dying of the self, the allowing of vulnerability and the transformation of independence to attachment through coupling, cooperation, and cocreation.

Orgasm is called the little death, because the male offers a portion of his life force. The female sacrifices her freedom as a self-directed, independent single unit. The dark fire of sexual passion transforms both into spiritually driven, cocreating forces.

Through their lovemaking they experience a moment of oneness, a transforming act that changes them both forever. Their molecules have been mixed. Their Emotional Bodies are intertwined, but so are the Spiritual and Mental bodies that exist in the aura surrounding their physical selves.

They may each forget or purposely put away from memory the occasion of their completion. However, it continues to exist as a change in the electromagnetic vibratory field that surrounds each.

If the outcome is positive, the individuals show signs of rejuvenation because there was an equal energy exchange. If the outcome is not balanced, each person is diminished. With the planetary burgundy ray of Pluto, there is no such thing as neutral reaction. It will transform, positively or negatively.

Eastern religions that infiltrated the Western world made millions of dollars teaching Americans to kill their desire. Americans feel guilty for being so creative, productive, and prosperous, yet we support or feed most of the countries that are professing the Eastern path to spiritual bliss. Their program of expecting nothing, desiring nothing, and doing nothing has produced nothing. The red and burgundy rays have stimulated only their sexual desires because the single most apparent result of their creative desire has been overpopulation.

Most of us think of passion in terms of animal lust, of loosening our straitjacket of controlled emotions to an unbridled outpouring of physical expression.

But passion is also the action of an individual directed toward any creative function. The desire of a poet to create reaches a vibrational rate of passion. The outpouring of a painter, sculptor, composer, inventor, writer, architect, etc. equals sexual passion's vibrational rate. In all instances it becomes a giving and a receiving. In order to receive, we must first give. This is an indisputable law of the Universe.

In the present age we have seen a pronounced emphasis on diseases of the life-giving organs resulting from the abuse of creative forces. The spread of AIDS and herpes has already begun to change some minds about promiscuity. The ancient knowledge and philosophies of Tantric Yoga and the Kundalini forces all deal with the transformation of the sexual urge toward physical union with another into the creative, spiritual union with the Universal Mind, Creator, God.

The Fire Opal from Mexico, being clear and pure and red, corresponds in every vibration to true passion. If this Opal is used in meditation, it will stimulate both the sexual and mental creative passions, discriminating between the two and directing the energy into the intended perfect balance.

There are various disturbances of the regenerative systems in women that can be attributed to negative mind-set that comes from imbalance. Feeling restricted often causes the pain that accompanies their monthly cycle. Domination by another person, or the attempt to dominate someone else, can cause constriction and pain near the ovaries.

Sterility can be caused by hatred, fear, or anxiety. The fallopian tubes may close tightly when there is some hidden hostility toward the mate. This same symptom can occur if strong parental threats concerning sex are carried over into marital relationships. These are examples of how the invisible bodies are affecting the physical activities. On the surface, these problems appear to be distinctly medical. When crystals are used in daily exercises the Emotional Body and the Mental Body are treated.

In the male, impotence can often be traced to childhood feelings of hostility toward the female, usually the mother. The prostate problems suffered by men can sometimes be traced to infidelity, either within the marriage or a close relationship. Sometimes the triangle is not reality but rather a mind function, such as occurs when a father-daughter relationship or a mother-son affection is so strong it negates the other parent.

There are crystals that will balance the chemicals of the yin-yang principle that have far-reaching effects on anyone using them sincerely. Time spent concentrating upon the vibration of the Red Garnet would bring about the perfect comprehension of the individual using it, relating to their male-female perfection within. For a man, his inner woman would develop, making his associations with the other half of the world population harmonious and pleasing. For a woman, her inner man would develop, vastly improving all her relationships and her understanding of her counterparts.

Pluto represents transformation or death and rebirth. The Garnet transmits the rays of Pluto into our bodies through the "power center of life." That is a thinking area of the actual mind system located in the generative organs. The use of the generative organs during our past and present evolution has been strictly on a material-physical level. We were commanded to create more of ourselves and to populate the Earth.

Pluto's ray-waves will transform that strictly physical life-giving power center into a spiritual life-giving power center. Let us say that we will learn the interaction of true love that gives life itself meaning.

The vibration arising from the Lapis Lazuli of this sexual geometry is the ability to raise love from the erotic level to the sensitive heart level. In the case of anyone who is "waiting" for love, this vibration will raise their awareness to the love that already exists. With a stimulated heart, they will be able to recognize and respond to that higher aspect of love—not discounting the sexual, but elevating the spirit of each.

To continually wish that my parents were different in their love for me, or that my children were different in their love for me, or that my lover was different in his love for me—is to constantly negate the love that DOES EXIST from them. To constantly be waiting in expectation for that one great love to envelop us and overcome all our disappointments is like holding our breath for a lifetime. It will only make us one of the "living" dead.

The pink ray, transmitted by the Rose Quartz, is a mutation and combination of the silver and red rays of the Moon and Mars respectively. As it enters the body through the thymus gland near the heart chakra, it is working in the "mind power center of love." The heart is a separate thinking entity. It has always been known and felt as such, and it truly is a mind power. The pink rays, working through the Rose Quartz in the heart area, can soften to gentleness the hardened, vigorous, demanding vibrations from Mars by the receptiveness of the Moon. Dictatorship and controlling love give way to tender response in soft love. Self is most in need of acceptance by Self; and this will lead to manifestation of love with others.

The Ruby stimulates the heart and works upon the "mind power center of love." As we have said, the heart thinks on its own. When this "mind in the heart" is stimulated by wearing and meditating with a Ruby, the red ray of devotion activates a new love understanding.

It is a simple commandment, yet we often miss the meaning of it: "Love thy neighbor *as thyself*." First and foremost our only chance of higher living is to love, honor, and appreciate the marvelous creation of our Self!

We must recognize our own value as replicas of the larger body of the Mother-Father Universal Body. Then we can begin to connect emotionally with love and understanding to others, all like ourselves, from whom we are now psychologically separated. In learning to totally accept ourselves, we learn to unconditionally accept our fellow travelers. This is the beginning of wisdom.

8/Healthy Animals and Plants

"Healing is based on rapport, suggestion . . . and an unknown energy."

—Dr. Phineas Quimby
Teacher of Mary Baker Eddy

▲▲▲

Because the crystals can have an effect on the electromagnetic field of every living thing (and everything has life), then of course we want to treat our great friends, the animals and the plants. So many of us have precious pets in the animal kingdom and daily enjoy our garden and house plants in a symbiotic exchange of love and energy! Psychologists have long known that the companionship of a pet can bring a new joy and self-acceptance to persons living alone or experiencing pain. The animal can also experience greater health through our loving care. This is a story that taught me how the crystals can treat animal infirmities. It also illustrates the answer to the often asked question: "Could this crystal healing be merely mind over matter or autosuggestion?"

One of my friends was introduced to a gentleman who had a longtime companion named Foxy, an aged Doberman. Foxy was elderly and crippled by arthritis, which made her a very harmless and gentle dog, not at all like the stereotyped watchdog. My friend gave the crystal (a five-inch cloudy Quartz) to the owner as an experiment, to see if a nonbeliever could actually clear the cloudiness from the Quartz by carrying and holding it.

After about six weeks I got a call from the man. Skeptically he told me, "I'm only calling because I know you're interested in these things." He went on to report that he indeed thought his crystal had become a bit more clear. Then he really surprised me with this story:

Healthy Animals

You know, I've been carrying that darn crystal around here for about six weeks, and I started to stroke Foxy with it while she's lyin' beside my chair. You know, she always lays there and I always pet her a lot while I'm readin'. My wife seemed to take to that crystal and she started layin' it in Foxy's bed at night. Foxy's been all crippled up for about two years and she hasn't even been able to take a walk up the hill for months. We've been takin' her to the vet and givin' her shots, just so she could walk at all. Well, when we took her to the vet this month, he couldn't believe how much better she was! She didn't have to have her cortisone for the first time in two years!

Now, you know I'm just tellin' you this 'cause I know you're interested in these things. Do you think that crystal could have had anything to do with Foxy's arthritis gettin' better?

We know the man wanted his dog to get better. The dog was old and the man had no actual expectations of her getting well, but he dearly loved her. This healing could have taken place in one of two ways or both: The crystal could have used the owner's electromagnetic brain waves and Emotional Body energy to magnify or transmit it to the dog (love is an energy). Or, the crystal, being a natural tool provided for us, could have transmitted invisible cosmic rays of healing and the Earth's healing energies to Foxy.

Whatever the reason, it will eventually be discovered by scientists who are investigating this in laboratories now. Until they prove it, there is one thing I have discovered: Unlike medicine or surgery, THE CRYSTALS CAN'T HURT.

I suggest that it might be very good for all our pets to have a small Quartz crystal attached to a collar in a safe and harmless way.

I'm convinced the possible applications are endless. Why not use crystals on our milk-producing cows, our egg-producing chickens, in our fish tanks, with our zoo animals, in the stalls with our horses, in kennels and animal hospitals? My origin and background being Texan, I rarely ask "Why?" and usually ask "Why not?"

> "The so-called 'circadian rhythms' of plants that respond to day and night by opening and closing their blossoms or leaves have been found to continue this pattern *even* when the light is artificially altered. This leads me to believe that all such rhythms are being forced on the organism (and possibly humans) by some unknown radiation factor in the Universe."
>
> —**M. de Mairan**
> French Royal Academy, 1729

▲▲▲

The Christmas Poinsettia Case

The Clear Quartz crystal, being the most abundant and therefore the least expensive, seems to be our most versatile friend. How good our Mother Earth is to us! I have a large collection of quality specimens from different areas around the U.S. and different countries in the world. I made a display on a table in my waiting room.

Several Christmases ago I went to a nursery and carefully chose three perfectly matched potted red poinsettias for my decorations in that room. I was also given a gift, a pink-blossomed poinsettia, which I placed with the others around the room. All had equal light (there are many large windows) and equal exposure to heat and drafts. I watered them equally, petting and speaking to each when I did this. That room also has daily instrumental music vibrations of a kind that I believe to be healthful for plants and humans.

One of the plants was nestled in the center of my Quartz

specimen collection. The others were not more than five to ten feet away in all directions.

Poinsettias are hardy houseplants and usually maintain their blossoms and leaves indoors for some time if properly cared for. They do have a limit, however, and will begin to fade after about two months, losing lower leaves.

All of the plants in the room began to do their usual fading and leaf dropping at about the same time . . . except the one in the Quartz collection. The others all stopped blooming after about three months and by four months had to have dead branches cut out. After five months two of the plants died, which is not unusual.

I was sorry to sacrifice the other plants, but when I realized what was happening, I chose to complete the experiment. I periodically moved the healthy plants and the Quartz collection together, rotating the position of the plants so that each one could have a time on the table where the Quartz was (maybe that table was a special place).

After eight months the two remaining plants were like distant cousins. The one with the Quartz collection was covered with red blossoms and bushy green leaves. The other plant was still green with no blossoms, but very tall and thin. I decided to conclude the experiment. I put a Quartz crystal about finger size in the dirt of the skinny cousin. You guessed it! There was a miraculous recovery, including more leaves and new blossoms.

The healthy plant has not stopped blooming in three years. The recovered plant has never quite caught up, but it's healthy.

Because of this discovery, I have treated all my outdoor blooming bushes to a healthy chunk of Quartz, buried halfway into the dirt at the base of the plant. I have also seen a difference in their growth and blooming activity.

You might want to experiment in this way.

I have heard other crystal teachers say that Quartz has an effect on machines also. I personally believe that some machines become like pets to us. For instance, a lot of people give a name to their automobile, motorcycle, or boat. I know a serious businessman who affectionately speaks to his car as "George." Somehow these machines take on personality.

My car has never been very well; she's had ailments ever since she was born. I have spent a lot of time and energy healing her. Now I am experimenting with a large chunk of Amethyst crystals on the front floor, as close to "Burgundy's" heart as I can place it. I also plan to try the suggestion of taping a small crystal to the gas line.

I've never thought of my refrigerator as a pet or given it a name, but it certainly is a member of the family! There are also some claims, which I am testing now, about cutting the electric bill by putting a Quartz in the refrigerator!

Part Three

THE HEALING COLOR CONNECTION: CRYSTALS AND THE PLANETS

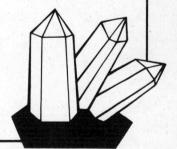

"The colors of nature have had their influence on us, and these influences are deep-seated in our physiological and psychological makeup."

—Dr. Max Lüscher

▲▲▲

There have been over two thousand minerals identified on Earth in different vibrations and states of development. Some are more mature than others. Some are more plentiful, others obscure. I use the criteria that the crystal or gem be readily available for use by the public. Mineral collectors are experts who may know of other healing gems that will fit these descriptions, but it would not be efficient to list crystals too expensive or obscure. The stones or minerals that I do *not* use in healing are lovely to look at, and sometimes to touch. I use the measurement of their durability taken from the scientific list of hardness called the Mohs' scale, in which all stones or minerals are measured on a scale from one to ten. I use only crystals that are 4½–5 hardness or more. I have tried using crystals that other writers claim are healing and have found them to be too soft. They crumble or break apart. I do not believe the crystals should die to heal us. When they cannot withstand the human vibration in daily use we need to respect their fragile beauty. An example is Fluorite, beautiful but too tender for use. There are other stones that duplicate vibrations of crystals I have listed here—but on a lower scale; for instance Citrine and Amber are a lower vibration of Topaz, so I do not list them.

The time when I was traveling to visit and to view the great gemological-mineralogical museums, studying the myths and legends of the jewels, was the most stimulating period of my research. Each crystal had a mystery to be solved. Tracing them through history, I reviewed their relationships with famous and infamous characters whose names we all know. I invite you to enjoy the adventure ahead and explore the crystal secrets for yourself. Be determined to add your own discoveries of the healing, powerful, and sweet energies you find in the crystals.

Reclaim the wisdom of the ancients with your own superconscious knowing.

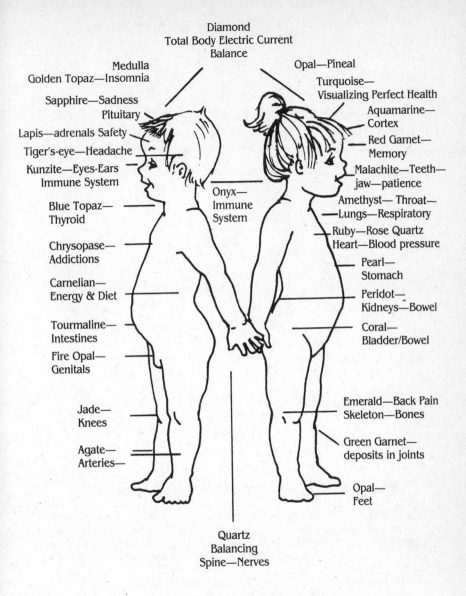

Diamond
Total Body Electric Current
Balance

Medulla
Golden Topaz—Insomnia

Opal—Pineal

Turquoise—
Visualizing Perfect Health

Sapphire—Sadness
Pituitary

Aquamarine—
Cortex

Lapis—adrenals Safety

Red Garnet—
Memory

Tiger's-eye—Headache

Kunzite—Eyes-Ears
Immune System

Malachite—Teeth—
jaw—patience

Blue Topaz—
Thyroid

Onyx—
Immune
System

Amethyst— Throat—
Lungs—Respiratory

Ruby—Rose Quartz
Heart—Blood pressure

Chrysopase—
Addictions

Pearl—
Stomach

Carnelian—
Energy & Diet

Peridot—
Kidneys—Bowel

Tourmaline—
Intestines

Coral—
Bladder/Bowel

Fire Opal—
Genitals

Jade—
Knees

Emerald—Back Pain
Skeleton—Bones

Agate—
Arteries—

Green Garnet—
deposits in joints

Opal—
Feet

Quartz
Balancing
Spine—Nerves

PHYSICAL AID WITH CRYSTALS

In order to use crystals in a general way, without knowing the invisible body that needs treatment, you may want to experiment with the crystals that have been suggested just for the physical body. There are many diverse opinions on this subject, and this illustration is very generalized, based on reports from my clients.

If you experience additional benefits, please write to me.

ASTROLOGICAL RULERSHIP OF THE HUMAN BODY

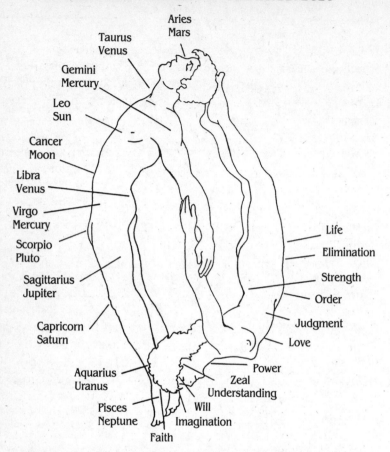

Aries
Mars

Taurus
Venus

Gemini
Mercury

Leo
Sun

Cancer
Moon

Libra
Venus

Virgo
Mercury

Scorpio
Pluto

Sagittarius
Jupiter

Capricorn
Saturn

Aquarius
Uranus

Pisces
Neptune

Faith

Will

Imagination

Understanding

Zeal

Power

Love

Judgment

Order

Strength

Elimination

Life

TWELVE AREAS OF MIND PENETRATED BY COSMIC RAYS

This illustration will help you to see where the mind power centers are on the human body. It is at these points on the electrical pathways or circuits (called meridians in acupuncture) that the cosmic color ray-wave vibrations of light transmitted by the planets enter our bodies. They are received and focused by using the proper crystal.

This same illustration also shows the ancient traditional astrological rulership that certain planets have over an assigned part of the body.

Even though the sun's rays enter into the body through the head at the power center of faith, it rules the heart. In the astrological chart of a heart disease patient, often the position of the Sun is negatively aspected. In medical astrology that would signal caution.

After you have chosen your crystal, find the gem chapter that explains the power center activated by your crystal, then check the illustration to see where it enters your body.

A *crystal* is a natural geometric formation. It has a uniform body with a geometric lattice. The varying properties of crystals, minerals, and gems (shape, color, vibration, hardness, etc.) are caused by the variations in the lattice structure.

Stones is the collective name for all solid constituents of the Earth's crust in the study of geology.

Minerals are the natural solid constituents of the Earth's crust in the study of minerology. Most minerals have definite crystal forms.

Gemstones is the collective name for all ornamental stones. Most gemstones are minerals, with few exceptions.

Jewels are every piece of personal ornament, i.e., jewelry. They can also refer to cut or faceted unset gemstones.

Rhinestones were originally small rounded quartz crystals found along the Rhine River of Europe. They were faceted and used for less expensive personal ornaments.

Lead crystal is glass.

GEM-RAY CONNECTION

Crystal (Gem)	Psychic Qualities	Health Factor	Color Ray & Planet
AGATE	acceptance, cooperation	strengthens immune system	Silver Ray, Moon
AMETHYST	purifying and clarifying thoughts	protects throat, lungs, and respiratory system, healing others	Violet Ray, Mercury
AQUAMARINE	anxiety relief, peace of mind	pineal gland, right brain, kidneys	Blue-Violet Ray, Venus
BLUE TOPAZ	calmness, hypertension relief	thyroid balancing down	Blue Ray, Uranus
CARNELIAN	thyroid balancing up, energy overcoming inertia	adrenal glands stimulation, laziness	Red Ray, Mars
CHRYSOPRASE	addictions, overindulgence	thyroid and diet control	Green Ray, Saturn
CORAL	self-sacrifice, willingness to serve "Whole"	elimination of bladder, bowel	Red Ray, Pluto
DIAMOND	abundance, prosperity (material and spiritual)	total body purifying, magnifying other gems	Multi-Ray, Sun
EMERALD	honesty, love to others, self-disclosure	skeleton, bones, spine, teeth	Green Ray, Saturn
FIRE OPAL	physical response, passion, physical awareness	genitals and reproductive system	Red Ray, Pluto
GARNET	mystery, past-life ailment	memory	Red Ray, Pluto
JADE	problem solving and detection	knees	Green Ray, Saturn
LAPIS LAZULI	courage, protection from psychic attack, safety, self-protection	right brain, hormone balancing down, negative thought forms, Kundalini	Blue Ray, Uranus
MALACHITE	patience, self-control	teeth	Green Ray, Saturn

ONYX	gathering information	feet	Silver Ray, Moon
OPAL	left brain, psychic awareness	pineal gland	White Ray, Neptune
PEARL	forgiveness, smoothing over an irritation	stomach	Silver Ray, Moon
PERIDOT	spiritual increasing	lower back, strength, elimination	Yellow-Green Ray, Jupiter
QUARTZ	awakening to cosmic forces	heart and spine "systems" balance	Multi-Ray, Sun
ROSE QUARTZ	gentleness	very mild cardiac stimulant and diuretic	Red Ray, Mars
RUBY	self-love, will to live	heart strength, blood pressure	Red Ray, Mars
SAPPHIRE	alertness, overcoming sadness	blood circulation, pituitary balancing	Blue-Indigo Ray, Uranus
SPODUMENE KUNZITE	unconditional love	eyes, ears	Violet Ray, Mercury, Venus
SUGILITE	eliminates fear-transformation, makes chaos bearable	stops runaway adrenaline rush and other involuntary physical body reactions	Violet and Burgundy Ray, Mercury and Pluto
TIGER'S-EYE	concentration, focusing energy	medulla (brain), headache relief	Brown-Yellow Ray, Jupiter
TOPAZ	joy, now awareness, optimism	pituitary station, vitamin-hormone balance	Yellow Ray, Jupiter
TOURMALINE	3 bodies balance (physical, mental, emotional, spiritual)	intestinal tract	Multi-Ray, Vulcan
TURQUOISE	ancient wisdom, creativity, imagination, courage to speak truth	seeing into the body parts	Blue Ray, Uranus

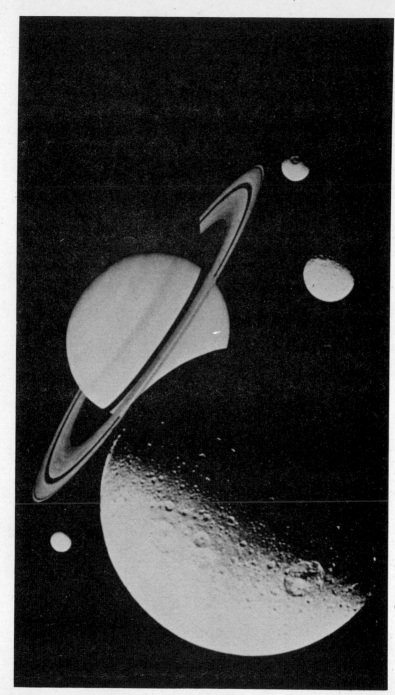

Saturn the great teacher is seen among his many moons. Ruler of rocks, minerals, and crystals, Saturn is sending us the green ray of truth and structure.

The Sun
Total Color Prism

DIAMOND • CLEAR QUARTZ CRYSTAL

"The pattern or organization of any biological system is part determined by its atomic physio-chemical components. Energy fields surround power and maintain every living system, from tiny plants to human beings."

—Dr. Harold Saxton Burr
Electrodynamic Theory of Life
Professor of Anatomy, Yale, 1935

▲▲▲

Of the cosmic rays that come to Earth from the twelve sources in our Universe, those from the Sun are the most powerful. Entering the body through the pineal gland, the third eye, they activate the mind power center of faith.

Humans have worshiped the Sun as "god" in every civilization since the beginning of history. We might say, "How primitive," but the indisputable fact remains that the Sun gives life to the Earth.

91

The Diamond, as the most highly evolved crystal on Earth, brings us the ray connection of the Sun. White light contains every color in the spectrum. It is the force behind life and the evolution of the universe. The brilliance of the white ray is so powerful that physically we cannot survive its strength if we are exposed to it too long.

All esoteric writings contain references to white and black because both contain all except each other. James Sturzaker, in his book *The Twelve Rays,* tells us that the white ray is expansion. It is interpreted as life-giving and life-saving. Like the Diamond, which is made of the most perfect element, carbon, it is the basic structure of all life and the most indestructible; it can only be destroyed by its own element. Heat, which creates the Diamond, also destroys it.

The gem-ray connection that is made by the transmission of the Sun through the Diamond is an unbreakable bond and a promise to us from our Mother-Father Creator. The rainbow that was a promise in the Talmudic history of the flood is created again and again by the Diamond.

The reflection of the Sun in the Diamond, with all the facets of life on Earth, is a constant reminder of the micro-cosm of the macro-cosm. Black and white, life and death, the message is faith and the belief that in the end, light always triumphs over darkness.

The Clear Crystal Quartz also receives and transmits the cosmic rays from the Sun as well as from the Moon and a small combination of the other rays. Like the Diamond, it is a multi-ray transmitter. The Diamond is the highest frequency, therefore it magnifies. The Clear Crystal Quartz merely transmits.

Affecting no specific area of the body or psyche, the Clear Quartz affects all to a degree. It does not enter the body at one point, but at all points. Somehow, the Clear Quartz crystal receives reflected rays from the center of the Earth as well as from the planets.

DIAMOND

CHEMICAL COMPOSITION: C (crystallized carbon)
CRYSTAL SYSTEM: Isometric (cubic)
WHITE RAY (total color prism)
PLANET: Sun
POWER CENTER OF FAITH
HEALTH FACTORS: Total body purifying
PSYCHIC QUALITIES: Material and spiritual abundance; prosperity

General Science

The Greeks called the Diamond *adamas*, which means "unconquerable." We derive our translation from that, because the Diamond is the hardest of all gems. It can only be cut with another Diamond. On the Mohs' scale of hardness, it is the only #10 gem.

Up to the 1700s, Diamonds were found in Borneo and India. These deposits now appear to be worked out. In 1775 the first Diamonds were found in Minas Gerais, Brazil, and South America. In 1867 the first Diamond was found in South Africa in the Orange River region.

There are also deposits in Siberia and the Ural Mountains of Russia. Almost a quarter of the Diamonds mined there are gem quality. In the United States small deposits have been found at several sites. The largest Diamond ever found in America, in Murfreesboro, Arkansas, weighed forty carats.

Only about twenty percent of all Diamonds mined are suitable for gems. The rest are called "unseen." These are also valuable as they are used in the production of almost every product we use.

Industry uses Diamond dust for grinding and cutting. Automobiles, bicycles, wires, screws, electrical equipment, refrigerators, toasters, radios, television, and light bulbs all depend on Diamond dies. Diamond drills are used by dentists and those who drill for oil in the Earth. Diamonds are used in rocketry and space exploration.

History, Myth, and Magic

Rough Diamonds were the playthings of children in Africa. It is said that when Europeans first traveled to Africa, they saw Diamonds in the leather pouches of witch doctors.

As the Diamond was found to be indestructible through all ages, it was fitting that knights should have them adorning their suits of armor and that monarchs would wear them in their crowns.

The most well-known use of Diamonds today is the engagement ring given to a bride by her groom. It is believed this was an English inspiration begun with the printing of old ballads in 1846. In one particular ballad, the princess gave a ring to her lover before he went to sea. The ring was set with seven Diamonds. While he was at sea, the Diamonds grew dim. He quickly returned, just in time to save her from a marriage the king would have forced upon her.

The Diamond has been given as a sign of trust, and as a long, strong, enduring promise of faithfulness, ever since.

Healing Secrets

The Diamond, being the purest of all gems, actually purifies the whole system of anyone who will consciously meditate with it. Although each gem can impart a certain benefit when in contact with the body, if the mind and spirit are not tuned in consciously to the powers that are available, they will only help to maintain a status quo.

Not everyone may own a Diamond, because the Diamond market is strictly controlled. This also excludes rough crystal Diamonds from the marketplace. However, those who are consciously striving to be on a balanced routine in life, and are aware of gem vibrations, will also make some sacrifice to own a Diamond, no matter how small. The vibration remains the same, even in the Diamond dust used for grinding wheels.

The Diamond is a magnifier of all the other crystal formulas. It is best to use it in partnership with a colored crystal.

The Sun, sending its ray-wave to the Diamond specifically, gives life to Earth. Everything that the Sun does for us is magnified by the Diamond. It increases all of our body mechanisms that are so perfectly designed and balanced.

It is possible to have fingers dripping with Diamonds yet die of debilitating disease. Ultimately, because we have free will, we make the decision to be healthy or to be healed. No crystal can force any activity within our body, mind, or spirit unless we consciously cooperate.

To have a small chip of the Diamond set with, or near, the colored crystal that affects the physical area needing protection would magnify the healing process.

Psychic Strengths

The "mind power center of faith" is located in the brain at the pineal gland. This is just above the ears and adjacent to the eyes, at the center of the brain. In all ancient writings, this is referred to as the "third eye."

Paracelsus, a German physician practicing in the 1500s, was also a powerful metaphysician. He believed the mind power center of faith could ultimately cure all disease.

An American physician, Dr. Phineas Quimby, who lived

and practiced in New England in the 1800s, was the inspired forerunner of new-age healing. He taught his patients to change their beliefs concerning illness and disease.

Dr. Quimby is credited with being the originator of the "mind cure," long before Sigmund Freud made history with psychoanalysis. Quimby's patients and historians recognized him as an American guru of mental and spiritual healing.

The "mind power center of faith," centered in the brain, is activated by meditation with the Diamond. It can bring about physical, emotional, and spiritual changes with a more efficient focus than we can achieve without it.

DIAMOND MEDITATION

Faith, as a mind power, is the basic vibration set up in the pineal gland by the Diamond. This psychic power is increased through meditation, so that we may receive what we desire and that which is good from the abundance of the Universe.

The metaphysical act of believing, and speaking the words aloud, is actually an active pulling together of physical atoms, like magnetism.

In all orthodox religions the word "faith" is used. It is the act of believing, even when the conscious mind cannot see the possibility. Jesus, beloved teacher and healer, said, "All things whatsoever ye pray and ask for, believe that ye receive them and ye shall have them."

Even the smallest Diamond chip, set with the colored crystal that affects the physical area needing protection, would magnify the healing. Use in daily meditation will:

1. Give the wearer a feeling of safety and security

2. Purify the whole body system
3. Increase the properties of all colored gems

Method

Lie down on the floor on your back, hold the Diamond in your palm, and gaze at it for one full minute.

Place the Diamond against the . . .

SOLAR PLEXUS (near waist): Cover with palm, repeat seven times . . . "This Diamond is vibrating power to me from the rays of the Sun."

HEART: Cover with palm, repeat seven times . . . "This Diamond is a long, strong bond between me and my Creators."

FOREHEAD ("third eye"): Cover with palm, repeat seven times . . . "This Diamond is daily increasing my faith in myself as a Creator."

CLEAR QUARTZ

CHEMICAL COMPOSITION: SiO_2 (silicon dioxide)
CRYSTAL SYSTEM: Hexagonal (trigonal)
WHITE RAY (total color prism)
PLANET: Sun
ENTERS THE BODY AT ALL POINTS
HEALTH FACTOR: Corrects imbalance anywhere in the body
PSYCHIC QUALITIES: Awakens Cosmic Consciousness

General Science

The word "quarz" is German; the word "crystal" is derived from the Greek word "krystallos," meaning ice.

The clear (rock) Crystal is one of the most plentiful specimens on Earth of the very large Quartz family. There are two varieties. One side of the Quartz family is found commonly growing in very well-formed individual crystals. This group is called macrocrystalline. The other members are found in beds of layers, amorphous growths, or large chunks where the crystals are not obvious to the naked eye. These are called microcrystalline.

Among the well-formed crystal group (Amethyst, Citrine, Smokey Quartz, Tiger's-eye, Hawk's-eye, Rose Quartz, and Clear Quartz), the Clear Quartz is the most abundant. It is found almost everywhere on Earth.

In the United States some of the most spectacular single crystals have been found in caves in Arkansas. The small, double-ended, very clear crystals found in Herkimer, New York, are often referred to as "Herkimer Diamonds" because they are so sparkling bright and appear as faceted gems.

Even though Quartz Crystal has a hardness of 7 on the Mohs' scale, no matter how it is cut or faceted, it doesn't seem to have enough sparkle to make it popular for jewelry. It used to be very popular in carvings and vases. It was also ground into a perfect sphere to be used in divination, or seeing into the future.

Years ago small Quartz pebbles, picked up on the banks of the Rhine River in Germany, were given the name "Rhinestones." Now, we make Rhinestones of glass for costumes and jewelry.

Quartz has very important characteristics that make it useful in industry. Under pressure, it produces heat; when heated, it produces electricity. It does not conduct electricity even in moisture. It reverses the plane of polarity as it absorbs light in different ways from different angles.

Every time you tune in your radio, the Quartz crystals inside, electrically oscillating (vibrating) at a fixed rate, keep the transmitters on their own wavelengths. The telephone company uses these crystals also, so that thousands of different messages can travel together but remain separate.

Rock crystal Quartz was ground into sheets that provided the first reading glasses and lenses for telescopes. The relative coolness of the Quartz kept it from overheating.

Glass cannot compare in any way to crystal Quartz—there is a totally different vibration. Quartz refracts the light doubly and glass does not. Don't be misled into buying glass crystal when you want Quartz.

History, Myth, and Magic

As this rock crystal contains 46% silicon and 53% oxygen, it was very reasonable to ancient chemists that it could be powdered and mixed with water to cure many ailments.

Dr. John Dee was an attending physician, astrologer, and friend of Queen Elizabeth of England (1558–1603). His most famous healing stone, a rock crystal Quartz, is still preserved in the Ashmolean Museum at Oxford, England.

Dr. William Gregory, Professor of Chemistry at the University of Edinburgh, Scotland, translated in 1856 the study of crystal magnetism by Professor Karl Baron von Reichenbach, *Researches on Magnetism, Electricity in Relation to the Vital Force,* which established that the "polar force resides in crystals." He addressed the occult side of his science by stating positively that "every crystal exerts a specific action on animal nerves."

Healing Secrets

Magnetism is very important in the human body and diagnosis. The blood is the key to diagnosis, and the chemical makeup of the blood includes iron, which makes up the coloring matter of red blood corpuscles. The amount of iron in the bile of the liver is also important (phosphate of iron). Chemical balance, between the ferric and oxygenic (i.e., magnetic) conditions of the blood, is necessary for mental and physical health. The magnetic charges that are present in the rock crystal Quartz pick up and detect any imbalance.

In matters of health, it is a transmitter of imbalance detected by magnetism anywhere in the body.

Psychic Strengths

Quartz crystal is remarkably powerful in sensitive persons. Since the "polar luminosity" is sent out from the ends of the crystal, it causes a contact to the human hand similar to iron adhering to magnet. When the crystal is laid in the palm of a sensitive, it causes an involuntary clasping or clenching, almost as a spasm of the fist. This brought to Professor Gregory's attention a fundamental force. Sensitive persons could feel this force in each crystal more easily with the lips. These same persons could charge the crystal with their own magnetic or electric current to heal, through the mouth or breath, as in blowing on the crystal.

Professor Gregory stated further that crystal gazing, or using a crystal to diagnose, was possible because "there streams from human eyes magnetism, projected from the lesser brain (cerebellum), when the gaze is fixed upon a given point." He credited the crystal with the greatest possible influx of celestial or terrestrial magnetism.

More recently Marcel Vogel, a senior scientist for IBM, after twenty-five years of study using clear crystal Quartz in communications systems, has discovered the psychic and healing qualities of the gem. He has retired from corporate life and is devoting his genius full-time to continued experimentation and personally demonstrating to physicians and nurses the diagnostic and healing use of the clear crystal Quartz.

CLEAR QUARTZ MEDITATION

Meditating with a Clear Quartz crystal affects all areas of the body and all aspects of the psyche.

Clear Quartz polarizes, centers, and grounds the physical body. It produces mental and emotional cosmic awareness.

Meditation with a Clear Quartz will awaken any skeptic to the forces of nature, the unseen actualities of the mental world, and the personal electric power of the individual.

Quartz is a beginning, gentle vibration for anyone new to the metaphysical exploration of the unseen world. It is also a spectacular tool for the advanced healer. Because it is not preprogrammed or limited, it awaits the needs of its owner.

If a beginner in crystallography wishes to use this gem, understand that its very general vibration will lead to a gradual understanding to which you will wish to add more specific gems as awareness is achieved.

Method

Lie down on the floor on your back. Hold the Clear Quartz crystal in your palm and gaze at it for one full minute.

Place the Quartz against the . . .

SOLAR PLEXUS (near waist): Cover with palm, repeat seven times . . . "This Crystal is transmitting energy from all the planets."

HEART: Cover with palm, repeat seven times . . . "This Crystal is vibrating to help me tune in to my place in the Cosmos."

FOREHEAD ("third eye"): Cover with palm, repeat seven times . . . "This Crystal is awakening my own Cosmic Consciousness."

Silver-White Ray
The Moon

PEARL ◆ AGATE ◆ ROSE QUARTZ ◆ OPAL

"There is an emanation from us, not magical or miraculous, but a subtle, invisible substance, capable of perception, which consciously or unconsciously magnetizes and influences every person and object with which we come in contact."

—D. D. Palmer
Founder of Chiropractic

▲▲▲

The Moon transmits on the silver rays of the cosmic current, radiating perfect peace and tranquillity. It promotes meditation and perfect contemplation. It also controls the invisible silver cord that is said to connect each of us to our original Cosmic Parents. In esoteric philosophy, this silver cord is our Universal umbilical, which disconnects from the body at death.

Silver rays affect the Opal, Onyx, Agate, Pearl, and Clear Quartz crystal as they vibrate and transmit separate frequencies, entering the body at separate power points determined by their individual chemistry.

The white ray is the cleansing ray . . . the outgoing ray. It helps us to gain victory over the self. The symbols of the white ray are the unicorn, white horse, or white bull spoken of in myth and in all ancient religions.

The Pearl directs the silver and white rays into the "Mind Power Center of Judgment" near, and surrounding, the stomach. From there it is "felt," judged, and used throughout the body, mind, and spirit.

The Moon represents our emotions with its placement in our horoscope. It also represents our birth mother. In a man's chart it represents the perfect woman for his mate. It denotes our place of sensitivity and vulnerability.

Rose Quartz and Opal are also transmitting Moon vibrations, but they will be discussed under their primary transmitting planets: Mars and Pluto for Rose Quartz, and Neptune for Opal.

PEARL

CHEMICAL COMPOSITION: Calcium carbonate + organic + water
CRYSTAL SYSTEM: Microcrystalline
SILVER RAY
PLANET: Moon
POWER CENTER OF JUDGMENT
HEALTH FACTOR: Stomach
PSYCHIC QUALITIES: Forgiveness, smoothing over an irritation

General Science

The Ruby is from the same "root" gem as the Sapphire, called "corundum," derived from the Sanskrit *kuruvinda*. The bright, clear red to pink color is caused by the element chromium replacing the aluminum of the Sapphire. Chromium causes a bright red fluorescence in the precious Ruby. A bit of ferric iron sometimes adds a slight orange cast to the red, or a slight amount of aluminum may give the red a small purplish glint.

Rubies are second in value only to Diamonds, being 9½ on the Mohs' scale of 1 to 10 in hardness. There are so few Rubies unflawed in anything over 5 carats that anything larger is more valuable than a Diamond of equal quality and size. The finest Rubies occur near Mogok, Burma, in crystals up to two inches in length. Cambodia, Thailand, Ceylon, India, Tanzania, and Australia are all sources. The latest finds have been in Norway and in the Ural Mountains of Russia. Small, pink cut Rubies are made from the pebbles gathered in streambeds of the Orient. Very few raw specimens ever leave the country of origin, as gem quality stones are immediately faceted for greater value.

History, Myth, and Magic

The name "ruby" comes from the Latin word *rubeus*, meaning the color red. In the oldest written language of the Hindus, Sanskrit, the Ruby was described as being "red as the lotus." It was also called the king of precious stones. They believed that an inextinguishable fire burned inside the gem. Modern testing has proven that it does indeed give off heat. Ruby was conferred the highest honor of being called a Brahman, the highest caste in the Hindu religion. They believed that owning a Brahman Ruby was a perfect protection against bad luck.

On the Mohs' scale of hardness, the Pearl measures 3–4, however, due to their compact molecular structure, they are very strong and difficult to crush.

Pearls are measured, or weighed, in grains or carats like other gems. This weight is multiplied by the going price for the particular color, size, or type of Pearl. In this way the Pearl market is similar to the Diamond market.

History, Myth, and Magic

In the South Kensington Geological Museum in London, there is, on display, the largest Pearl ever reported. It weighs 450 carats (1,800 grains). Pearls have been used for adornment and have been considered valuable gems for at least six thousand years.

Records show that the Chinese had a very successful Pearl trade as early as 2500 B.C. The Chinese may have been the first to think of culturing Pearls. They began to place small lead sculptures of Buddha inside the shells of mollusks so they could be coated with the Pearl nacre.

Healing Secrets

In the seventeenth century, when powdered gems and crystals were prescribed to be taken internally, Pearls were given to cure tuberculosis or consumption. The plague, weak eyes, old age, and nervousness were also treated with the use of Pearls. Cleopatra put Pearls in vinegar to cure upset stomach. Paracelsus mentioned the dissolving of Pearls in lemon juice or vinegar to kill the acids of the stomach.

Wearing of Pearl, and meditating with it, can help to focus the cosmic Moon ray. We no longer crush or dissolve Pearls to take internally, for we have evolved to a higher understanding of the vibrations of crystals and how they can affect our bodies. This sea-born microcrystalline transmitter can have a physical effect on any irritation anywhere in the body, but especially in the liquid-related areas that are alternately regulated by the Moon rays.

Psychic Strengths

The Moon also rules the emotions of Earth's residents. The Moon is very close to Earth and we feel its direct effect continuously in the tides of Earth waters. These waters make up sixty percent of our bodies—including the brain. The mental faculties, or emotional moods, of all of us somehow relate to our physical responses to the cosmic rays that are constantly falling upon us like dew . . . unseen. The vibration of the Pearl, in transmitting the Moon's rays to our psyche, is to help us to smooth over irritations.

PEARL MEDITATION

The Pearl represents the Moon, ruler of Cancer, which is the sign of the zodiac attributed to the stomach.

The Moon rules the oceans and waters of the Earth where Pearls are born. The very process of Pearl formation is through an initial irritation in which liquid secretions smooth and soothe the irritated area.

Jesus spoke of Pearls as words of wisdom and ordered his disciples not to treat them lightly or to waste their knowledge on those who were not ready to hear.

If you are ready to allow the Cosmic Current to flow through you as it is meant to do and feel strongly attracted to Pearls, they will aid you. Born in the soothing sea, they continually carry that vibration. Use them to:

1. Smooth over an irritation
2. Increase perfect contemplation
3. Soothe the stomach

Method

Lie down on the floor on your back. Hold the Pearl in your palm and gaze at it for one full minute.

Place the Pearl(s) against the . . .

SOLAR PLEXUS (near waist): Cover with palm, repeat seven times . . . "These Pearls are vibrating to smooth over this irritation in my life."

HEART: Cover with palm, repeat seven times . . . "These Pearls are vibrating to increase my perfect contemplation."

FOREHEAD ("third eye"): Cover with palm, repeat seven times . . . "These Pearls are vibrating to soothe my judgment center."

AGATE

CRYSTAL COMPOSITION: SiO_2 (silicon dioxide)
CRYSTAL SYSTEM: Hexagonal (trigonal) microcrystalline
SILVER RAY
PLANET: Moon
POWER CENTER OF LIFE
HEALTH FACTORS: Strengthens immune system
PSYCHIC QUALITIES: Acceptance, cooperation

General Science

Another of the great family of Quartz, this special cousin is named for the river "Achates" on the island of Sicily. The Romans probably found Agates here in antiquity.

The most common forms of Agate are nodules or geodes, formed as liquids seep into hardened bubble cavities in volcanic rock. As different glassy, sandy, or liquid acids flow in and harden, they form different-colored layers. The first layer inside the cavity is usually the thickest, gray or white in color. It is called chalcedony. The next and alternate layers can be red, pink, brown, or golden.

If these alternating layers completely fill the cavity, when sliced open, it can give the bull's-eye effect. If there is a space left open in the center not filled with Agate mass, clear, small crystals of Quartz may form. This is called a geode. Amethyst, Smokey Quartz, Citrine, Hematite, etc. are found in this symbiotic formation. These cavities may reach huge proportions as in the case of lava flowing over prehistoric trees. When the tree decays, it leaves a large hollow to fill with Agate and its siblings.

All Agates measure a hardness of 7 on the Mohs' scale of 1 to 10.

Agate is rarely faceted. It is most commonly polished, domed or rounded (en cabochon), and used in jewelry or carved as small vessels.

History, Myth, and Magic

In Japanese graves dating from 10 B.C., curious amulets of carved Agate, called magatama, have been found. The combination of two magatama form the Chinese symbol for yin and yang—the masculine-feminine polarity principle. This insignia is still very prominent in Korea, Japan, and China.

In East India and Arabia, the polished Agate showing concentric circles was called the "eye agate." It was often used in the eyes of idols and was worn as an important amulet against the "evil eye."

A Catholic priest had some curious revelations in 1709. His sketches of an airplane, or flying machine, were published in Vienna along with a description of the use of Agate. Over the metal grillwork, at the top, were attached Agates that, when heated by the Sun, would become magnetic and cause the ship to rise. He actually may have been seeing far into the future, for Agate is a form of Quartz that is now being used in many industrial and power-producing designs.

In the *Natural History of Precious Stones* by King, in London, 1865, he quotes ancient Greek poetry as describing the Agate as a man's amulet for love to assure him of a woman's love.

Healing Secrets

When something becomes crystallized, it hardens. There are various areas in the body that are troubled by hardening, such as the arteries. Hardening of the arteries to the head can bring loss of memory and senility. In any other areas of the body, loss of circulation causes loss of function.

The Agate has a vibration to flush out and decrystallize areas that are affected. Kidney stones and gallstones can be disintegrated and flushed out by daily meditation with the Agate and wearing or carrying it constantly. Calcium, or salt crystal deposits, common in bursitis and arthritis, can also be broken up and flushed out of joints.

Psychic Strengths

When the thinking or belief systems are crystallized or hardened, they affect the whole body and personality. The Agate has a vibration to break up rigid thought forms. We make all the choices in every area of our lives. If we believe that we are victims of outside forces over which we have no control, our thinking is incomplete, rigid, and becomes a logjam that needs blasting.

AGATE MEDITATION

The Agate, one of the most common stones on Earth, is available to everyone to aid in transmitting the vibrations that will break up crystallized patterns and help transform themselves into accepting, adapting, and becoming new.

Method

Lie down on the floor on your back. Hold the Agate in your palm and gaze at it for one full minute.

Place the Agate against the . . .

SOLAR PLEXUS (near waist): Cover with palm, repeat seven times . . . "This Agate is vibrating to break up my rigid, outworn belief systems."

HEART: Cover with palm, repeat seven times . . . "This Agate is vibrating to help me adapt and cooperate with changing forces in my life."

FOREHEAD ("third eye"): Cover with palm, repeat seven times . . . "This Agate is vibrating to help me transform myself for the new world."

Mars and Pluto
The Red Ray

CARNELIAN ◆ CORAL ◆ FIRE OPAL ◆ RED GARNET ◆ RUBY ◆ ROSE QUARTZ

"The major shift in human evolution is from behaving like an animal struggling to survive to behaving like an animal choosing to evolve."

—Dr. Jonas Salk

▲▲▲

In all ancient esoteric writing, the color vibration of Mars is red. Astrologically, the red ray-wave issues from Mars, striking Earth and penetrating humans through the head and heart, giving energy, fire, and assertiveness to the races toward survival and evolution.

The fiery, assertive red ray-waves have given us, as Earth's inhabitants, the energy and vital consciousness toward forward movements of evolution, necessary not only to ensure survival, but also to sustain excited interest in living. At the beginning of every new Earth cycle is the Aries-Mars red ray energy.

The red ray or color vibration stimulates every new cycle. The red ray coursing through the Cosmic Universal Body of the Mother-Father creator represents our desire to create.

Modern technology observes and reflects this gem-ray connection, as the most potent new-age tool, the laser, is focused and activated through a Ruby. This miraculous, invisible ray-wave can microscopically cut the retina of an eye or powerfully cut through thick steel.

The planets Mars and Pluto both use the red ray as it enters the human body through the sacral chakra, located at the base of the spine or generative organs, known as the "mind power center of life."

Pluto, ruling the eighth house of the zodiac, is a very unusual planet. Its orbit is longer than that of any other planet of our galaxy, with an angle of ellipse that is in a numeric vibration different from all others. Pluto revolves around the Sun from west to east, taking 250 years to do so. In 1989 it will be at its nearest position to the Earth. From 1978 until 1999, Pluto will be nearer to the Sun than Neptune. During that time, the consciousness of all humanity will be increased.

Esoteric philosophers accept that humanity is being notified by the ray-waves of Pluto that we must learn self-knowledge. The activity of interpersonal relationships with close peers is to be a mirror for us.

Pluto affects the relationships of love between male and female but also includes all the primal feelings toward siblings and parents. The anxieties, jealousies, and other family dynamics that linger in our psyches for decades make us bitter, angry, and ill.

The planet Pluto is constantly transmitting a very high vibration that is not consciously felt by the masses. It is a continuous call to the spirit to surrender the self-destructive ideas, beliefs, and actions that so subtly sabotage our daily happiness and health.

Pluto is the planet of elimination, renewal, and regeneration. Its ray enters the body at the base of the spine where we sit. When we "sit" on a situation, doing nothing, it crystallizes.

Pluto stays up to twelve years in the same sign, causing its rays to affect whole generations. To show some of the ways in which Pluto's vibration has affected Earth, let's look at some of its transits since its discovery in 1930.

During its transit through Cancer, 1932–1945, Hitler rose to power and tremendous explosions shook the world in Japan and Germany. These two nations were transformed and reborn to financial superiority worldwide.

As Pluto moved through Leo and Virgo, in its next twelve-year transit, exciting transformations took place in communications and health care. Television provided a window whereby we could examine each other's private life. In health care the vitality of Dr. Jonas Salk's creation of the polio vaccine almost eliminated a life-threatening disease. The transit through Libra, designating partnership and marriage, saw the complete breakdown of the institution of marriage with the highest divorce rate in history. The rebuilding of the structure was evidenced as mothers and fathers switched roles.

The movement toward equality of the sexes and the falling away of outmoded, crystallized belief systems were forced by Pluto's rays. In Greek mythology, Pluto is often depicted holding a pitchfork, prodding someone in their sacral seat!

As Pluto enters Scorpio, where it will remain until November 10, 1995, we are seeing, as predicted by one of America's foremost astrologers, Marc Edmund Jones, that, "This cycle marks the overall and complete revolution of just about everything on the globe."

Scorpio rules joint money-accounts, sex, and mystical occult forces. It expresses itself passionately, secretly, and penetratingly. The alarming rate of sexually transmitted disease, such as Acquired Immune Deficiency Syndrome (AIDS), is one phase of Pluto in Scorpio.

This transit is especially strong because Pluto is the natural ruler of Scorpio. Both the planet and the sign represent death or transformation. Because of this, as well as the penetration of the unknown forces of nature attributed to Scorpio, the battle against AIDS will most likely uncover miraculous secrets of nature.

The other dynamic vibration that we can expect to affect us all is the deep probing of the mind into matters of spirit. Metaphysics will become a common study along with language, history, and mathematics. The whole planet will be affected as we each realize our part in the Universe and our personal power of mind.

The Indigo-Burgundy Ray

During certain climatic times around Earth, we are blessed with the visible rays contained within the rainbow. At this point in human physical evolution, our sight can discern seven rays. The one least mentioned is the indigo ray, which is an overlapping of the blue and violet rays. Crystal gems that transmit or trap the indigo ray may actually be receiving from Mercury and Uranus. The other possibility is that the indigo ray is actually from another source that is not known to us as an actual planet, or that its source planet is not in our solar system.

There are gem crystals that appear to transmit two rays. The Kunzite traps both blue and violet rays, as does Tanzanite and sometimes Alexandrite.

In many cases the blue ray and the indigo ray may be interchanging, only the indigo is more intensified.

Certain types of Red Garnet transmit the indigo-burgundy ray.

The Red Garnet and the Fire Opal are also discussed as two of the Love Crystals in Chapter 7, Crystals and the Yin-Yang Principle.

CARNELIAN-CORNELIAN

CHEMICAL COMPOSITION: SiO_2 (silicon dioxide)
CRYSTAL SYSTEM: Hexagonal (trigonal)
RED RAY
PLANET: Mars
POWER CENTER OF STRENGTH
HEALTH FACTORS: Stimulates adrenal glands, thyroid balancing up
PSYCHIC QUALITIES: Laziness, energy overcoming inertia

General Science

Carnelian-Cornelian is another of the family of Quartz, distinguished by the ancients from the various other varieties of Quartz such as "chalcedony" or "sard." The modern name is derived from the cornel cherry. The rusty red color is from iron oxide inclusions. It is one of the many microcrystalline quartzes, not growing in visible crystals or points, but in masses or beds.

The best quality is from India. As all other quartzes, the hardness on a scale of 1 to 10 is 7. Most Carnelian on the market today is Agate, dyed with ferrous nitrate solution, coming from Brazil and Uruguay.

History, Myth, and Magic

In many Latin gem treatises, the Carnelian is described as amulets inscribed with Arabic prayers. In these prayers, the stone is called upon to protect the wearer from evil or "tricks of the devil."

There is a legend that Muhammad wore a Carnelian ring, carved with the inscription, "The slave Abraham, relying on the merciful God." Napoleon, the great conqueror, somehow came to own this while in Egypt and wore it on his watch chain. He later gave it to Napoleon III, the Prince Imperial, who always wore it around his neck. He was killed by Zulus in South Africa. They stripped his body and the precious amulet was never recovered.

An Armenian writer in the 1600s wrote, "No man who wore a Carnelian was ever found in a collapsed house or beneath a fallen wall." Could this mean earthquake protection?

Healing Secrets

The Carnelian is a stimulant. It increases the thyroid and adrenal output. It increases deep breathing, which oxygenates the blood. It slightly increases the heart rate and can be used to revive from fainting or emotional shock. Carnelian causes the craving for proper nutrition, which is beneficial to obese or underweight individuals.

Psychic Strengths

Carnelian is the cosmic "kick in the pants." Its vibration is for energy and action in both body and mind. Lethargy or laziness are products of malnutrition—both of the body and of the brain. Boredom, lack of mental stimulation, and lack of proper nutrients are self-destructive tendencies that can be overcome with the stepped-up vibration of the Carnelian.

CARNELIAN MEDITATION

If the Carnelian is worn daily and actively used in meditation, it will increase the overall energy level as it transmits the stimulating Martian ray. Carnelian:

1. Promotes physical action
2. Encourages mental activity
3. Overcomes laziness or lethargy

Method

Lie down on the floor on your back. Hold the Carnelian in your palm and gaze at it for one full minute.

Place the Carnelian against the . . .

SOLAR PLEXUS (near waist): Cover with palm, repeat seven times . . . "This Carnelian is vibrating to give me energy and enthusiasm."

HEART: Cover with palm, repeat seven times . . . "This Carnelian is vibrating to promote physical action."

FOREHEAD ("third eye"): Cover with palm, repeat seven times . . . "This Carnelian is encouraging mental activity."

CORAL

CHEMICAL COMPOSITION: $CaCO_3$ (calcium carbonate, + magnesia and organic)
CRYSTAL SYSTEM: Hexagonal: Microcrystalline
RED RAY
PLANET: Pluto and Mars
POWER CENTER OF LIFE
HEALTH FACTORS: Elimination of bladder, bowels
PSYCHIC QUALITIES: Self-sacrifice, willingness to serve the "Whole"

General Science

Coral, as a gem, is formed differently from other precious crystals. It is formed in water by living organisms that fuse together and produce a calcium skeleton by their secretions. They appear to grow as small trees with bare branches.

Coral is very soft. On a hardness scale of 1 to 10, it measures only 3½.

Coral beds are worked systematically much like Pearl beds. Divers take the Coral only every tenth year. Some commercial Coral is harvested by dragging nets across the seabed, but this method destroys much valuable material.

The main trading center for Coral is in Torre del Greco, south of Naples, Italy. Some of the loveliest carved cameo pieces come from Italy, but Japan and China are also very productive in small carvings.

The most valuable color in the United States is oxblood, but in Japan it is pink.

History, Myth, and Magic

Coral has a long geological history. Fossils are found in rocks 400 million years old. There are two states in the

U.S. where fossil Coral has been found, Iowa and Ohio.

In Turin, Italy, in 1515, Albertus Magnus published his book on the secrets of healing in which he claimed that Coral would stop the bleeding of a wound. He also gave it psychological powers over madness.

One of the most costly Chinese amulets of the nineteenth century included five gems representing five deities, one of which was Coral, representing the "god of the sea" (or the element water). This amulet was suspended at the entrance to the home to protect against harm from the elements.

The American Indians incorporated Coral into their ceremonies and jewelry soon after the descendants of Christopher Columbus began trading with the eastern natives.

Alfred Tozzer studied Navajo ceremonies in the early 1900s. He noted that they used Coral to decorate the four rain-making gods in their ceremonial sand paintings.

Healing Secrets

Paracelsus (1493–1541), in his writings on gems and healing, was known to mix as many as thirty-four ingredients into a prescription, including Coral.

The red and the pink Coral both correspond to the "Mind Power Center of Life," described by Catherine Ponder. This power center is located in the generative organs. All diseases of these organs can be improved and/or cured by the wearing of Coral and by faithfully meditating with it daily.

The action of the Coral, as it builds itself slowly into a calcite substance by self-sacrifice and regeneration, correlates to that in our own bodies as we concentrate on healthy organs.

Water is one of the strongest and most powerful elements on Earth. The pressure (or stress) that is present in the oceans is equal to the pressures of the oceans of air (or atmospheres) in the space surrounding Earth. These pressures hold things together (gravity) and also hold things apart (repulsion).

Somewhere, within the water, there are patterns or veins invisible to the human eye that determine the growth patterns of the Corals.

This mysterious correspondence is brought about by the distant vibration of the planet Pluto. It rules the water sign of Scorpio and represents the generative and regenerative forces in the Universe and in humans.

The generative organs of the male and female human are constantly dealing with life-producing fluids.

The Coral corresponds to this portion of the physical body and can aid in the disintegration of destructive cells and the rebuilding of healthy cells.

Psychic Strengths

Psychic qualities inherent in the Coral are basically focused on the destruction of negatives—or portions of the psyche that have produced nontruth. This usually involves blaming someone else for results in our own life—or for any form of unfaithfulness that we take part in. These negatives can be regenerated by the conscious knowledge and effort of an individual in using the Coral as a tool to transmit new vibrations of thought from the cosmic current.

The tiny polyps that begin as living organisms in the water (much as we began billions of years ago) cling together and attract others. As they live in this symbiotic relationship, they secrete calcium, which solidifies. They die to produce this beautiful stone tree.

The parallel that takes place in our psyche as we use the Coral is that we begin to die to untruth, and we rebuild something valuable by taking full responsibility for our physical health—as well as spiritual health.

CORAL MEDITATION

All diseases of the generative organs can be improved and/ or cured by meditating with Coral daily.

Transmitting Pluto's rays, Coral sends a continuous call to the spirit to give up and let go of self-destructive ideas, beliefs, and actions that are subtly sabotaging our daily happiness.

The misunderstanding or abuse of sexual, creative power is mysterious to us. We can only experience the fulfillment of unity when we finally die to ourselves and totally surrender our will to control another.

Coral reaches down into the fluids of the body to stimulate the sacrifice of the self (willful ego), which is fearful of losing control in both the physical sexual encounter and the emotional love encounter.

Pluto vibrating through the Coral not only affects the relationships of love between male and female. It also includes all primal feelings toward siblings and parents, destroying and rebuilding the anxieties and jealousies that linger in our psyches for decades, making us angry, bitter, and ill.

Faithfully carrying or wearing Coral will:
1. Promote willingness to surrender willful ego
2. Encourage cooperative effort
3. Resurrect heart love
4. Regenerate diseased reproductive organs

Method

Lie down on the floor on your back. Hold the Coral in your palm and gaze at it for one full minute.

Place the Coral against the . . .
SOLAR PLEXUS (near waist): Cover with palm, repeat seven times . . . "This Coral is vibrating to help me surrender my old resentments and fears."
HEART: Cover with palm, repeat seven times . . . "This Coral is vibrating to help me cooperate in new-age collective efforts."
FOREHEAD ("third eye"): Cover with palm, repeat seven times . . . "This coral is vibrating to resurrect my heart love."

FIRE OPAL

CHEMICAL COMPOSITION: SiO_2 Hyalite
RED RAY
PLANET: Mars and Pluto
POWER CENTER OF LOVE
HEALTH FACTORS: Genitals and reproductive system
PSYCHIC QUALITIES: Physical response, passion, physical awareness

General Science

The Fire Opal is unto itself the most pure message of any gem. Being clear and pure and red, it corresponds in every vibration to true passion. If this Opal is used in meditation, it will stimulate both the sexual and mental creative passions. Like the other precious Opals, it will discriminate between the two and direct the energy into the intended perfect balance.

It is an established understanding that both famous and infamous individuals operated on basic, passionate energy levels. The outcome of their actions depended on channeling that passion into creative activity other than sex, therefore, sexual activity was in perfect balance with creative activity. If one overtakes the other, the balance is broken and the life suffers. Truly successful humankind is passionate about living, giving, and growing upward and forward. The thrust in human sexual passion is upward and forward. The natural motion of the Universe, expressed in the natural motion of satisfaction, gives the most natural reward.

The color red has always symbolized passion. The fact that the Fire Opal is not a complete geometric formula as all other red gems are guarantees its distinct nature. The tiny spheres recently discovered in the Opal structure are again a distinct pattern special to the Opal. In the black or white Opal, the variety of all colors combined in changing fires denotes that many messages can be heard (received) and transmitted. In the Fire Opal, the same is true for only one message. The message is passion, but the vibration is passion on all levels. The tiny spheres or building blocks that make up these Opals are symbolic of the sphere of the Earth with its varieties, and of the unending circle that makes our lives, deaths, and rebirths in the Universe. From the Creators, through the cycle, and back to the Creators is a full circle. We give of our passionate self, to be received by others and given back to us.

FIRE OPAL MEDITATION

The Fire Opal offers the purest vibrational message of any gem—passion!

Most of us equate passion to sexual excitement and tend to think of it in terms of pure animal lust. The giving we do in a state of passion, however, is total surrender of the self. What we gain is the elated state of true self-satisfaction.

The message is passion on all levels. If the Fire Opal is used in meditation, it will stimulate both sexual and mental creative passions, discriminating between the two, directing energy into the intended perfect balance.

History remembers famous and infamous individuals who operated on a basic energy that was certainly passionate. The outcome of their actions depended on channeling that passion into creativity other than sex. If one overtakes the other, the balance is broken and the life suffers.

In a passionate state we are most pure and most like our Creators, in whose passion we were conceived. Meditating with the Fire Opal will:

1. Stimulate excitement with life
2. Increase sexual passion
3. Empower surrender of the self
4. Activate creativity and adrenals

Method

Lie down on the floor on your back. Hold the Fire Opal in your palm and gaze at it for one full minute.

Place the Fire Opal against the . . .

SOLAR PLEXUS (near waist): Cover with palm, repeat seven times . . . "This Fire Opal is vibrating to increase my passion for life with excitement."

HEART: Cover with palm, repeat seven times . . . "This Fire Opal is vibrating to give me power through the complete surrender of my self."

FOREHEAD ("third eye"): Cover with palm, repeat seven times . . . "This Fire Opal is vibrating to stimulate my creative forces."

RED GARNET

(Almandite variety, precious)
CHEMICAL COMPOSITION: $Fe_3Al_2(SiO_4)_3$ (silicate ion)
CRYSTAL SYSTEM: Cubic or isometric
RED RAY
PLANET: Pluto
POWER CENTER OF LIFE
HEALTH FACTOR: All diseases of the regenerative organs, memory
PSYCHIC QUALITIES: Mystery, past-life ailment

General Science

The name Garnet is from the Latin *granutus*, meaning "like a grain." This comes directly from the pomegranate—the seeds of which resemble the Almandite Garnet.

There are six varieties of Garnet—the most commonly recognized being the Almandite, because it's a very dark red, brownish-red, or purplish-red color. It measures 7½ on the Mohs' scale of hardness from 1 to 10.

Garnet is found in many places including British Columbia, Alaska, Connecticut, Pennsylvania, Michigan, Idaho, Colorado. The best gems are from India, Africa, and Madagascar. The common elements that give the Almandite

Garnet its color are iron and aluminum. The crystals are formed of silicate and oxygen. Seen in the raw, the Garnet appears as though it had already been faceted. The faces of the crystals are easily recognized if they are found growing in rocks. They are common constituents of sand and are gathered as small pebbles in streams and riverbeds by the natives in India and Africa. The most precious crystals have been found in Hungary.

History, Myth, and Magic

In 1905, a necklace dating from 3500 B.C. was found in Egypt about the neck of a young male's mummified body. It contained many Almandite Garnets, Turquoise, and Amethyst. It so resembled the jewelry from the early graves of American Indians found in Arizona and New Mexico that it led to further speculation by historians and anthropologists that there is a definite link between the two peoples.

In 1892, on the Kashmir frontier, the British were astonished when a rebellious tribe of Hunzas fought them off with bullets made of Garnets. Many of these precious missiles have been preserved.

Garnets have been found in ancient Anglo-Saxon and Celtic jeweled armor. The chest protectors and girdles of metal were often inlaid with Garnet.

Pliny, in his treatise on gems some 2,500 years ago, noted that when he visited Alabanda, the ancient Persian city, he saw pint-size vessels cut from Garnet. These were probably large and common stones, lacking luster or quality.

One of the gems used by scientists to analyze the age of the Earth and its evolution, the Garnet is able to withstand enormous heat, up to 1400 degrees Fahrenheit. It was originally formed up to fifty miles beneath the Earth's crust. Because of this, the presence of red Garnet is indicative of the possibility of diamonds nearby.

Contemporary technology has discovered that the Garnet is so responsive to temperature that by warming or cooling it only a degree or two, it will reverse its polarity. This neat trick gives it the ability to store information in computer memory cells.

Healing Secrets

The Garnet transmits the rays of Pluto into our bodies through the "Mind Power Center of Life," the thinking area of the actual mind system located in the generative organs. The portion of the brain whose physiological activity affects the generative organs has always been thought to be the pituitary gland, as it distributes hormones. Now scientists are discovering that the hypothalamus at the base of the brain is actually directing the pituitary during arousal or desire.

The present age is seeing a definite accent on diseases of the life-giving organs caused by the misuse of the "Mind Power Center of Life." Garnet, used in healing this area of the physical body, can be directed toward any illness, for it vibrates the regeneration or transformation of the cell. The most effective healing for all diseases of the regenerative organs in particular would be through the Garnet.

In healing oneself or another, the Garnet is best used in full sunlight near the affected areas. If sunlight is not available, then incandescent light will substitute.

The ray-wave of Pluto, entering the brain through the hypothalamus and descending to the generative organs, can be used constructively to heal sexually related negative mind-set psychosomatic diseases such as sterility and impotence. By both physical application of a Garnet, and meditation daily with the Garnet, the hypothalamus will act upon the body.

Psychic Strengths

In transmitting the vibrations from Pluto, the Garnet becomes a transformer. It is both positive and negative balance—the yin-yang. In the positive it eliminates tension; in the negative it destroys old forms. In both these instances the Garnet can use the planet's energy to aid the transforming abilities of psychic healers. Pluto is the force that transforms the atomic structure of life. The Garnet is used to break down psychological blocks that prevent evolutionary growth. The Garnet works underground in our memory banks. Eventually it forces things out into the light. It is a very mysterious vibration that brings about the death of old, misbegotten thoughts and thought forms—the enemies of rebirth in our thinking through transforming the information.

We have many useful items and many self-destructive items locked within the vaults of our brain. On occasion, past remembrances are negative to our present life and are actually sabotaging our daily success. At other times, we need to recall successful experience and useful knowledge to activate our creativity. Releasing positive or negative thought forms is limited to only those that will be beneficial to the holder. Psychiatric therapy can take years to uncover what the vibration of the Garnet can reveal when used properly and with good intentions.

The double refraction of light in this gem gives off a double-coded message. The double element of iron-aluminum further contributes to this double meaning.

Aluminum is always found as a partner with other elements. It is silvery, lightweight, feminine, and cooperative in adjusting to change in itself and is very resistant to personal breakdown due to outside forces. In all metaphysical thought, especially astrology, the Moon is considered feminine.

Here we have a classic example of the dual polarity working in nature. Iron, the heavy, strong, masculine vibration, is vital to life. It can be formed and will unite with others, but it is susceptible to breakdown and disintegration from certain outside forces.

Wear a Garnet, meditate with it seven minutes daily if you need to improve male-female balance and transformation. The Garnet also stimulates the individual to look more deeply and with serious intent into the double or occult meanings of life, religions, philosophies, and metaphysics.

RED GARNET MEDITATION

Used in healing the physical body, the Garnet can be directed toward any illness. Because it vibrates the regeneration or transformation of the cell, it is most effective healing all diseases of the regenerative organs.

There are various disturbances of the regenerative systems that can be attributed to emotional or mind-set negativity. Feeling restricted often causes the pain that accompanies the monthly cycle of a female. Sterility can be caused by hatred, fear, or anxiety.

The ray-wave of Pluto entering the brain through the hypothalamus and descending to the generative organs can be used constructively to heal these and other real but psychosomatically caused diseases.

Working underground in our memory banks, Garnet is also used to break down psychological blocks that prevent evolutionary growth, eventually forcing things out into the light.

In healing oneself or another, the Garnet is best used in full sunlight near the affected areas. If sunlight is not available, incandescent light will substitute.

Meditation with the red Garnet will accomplish the following:

1. Open the memory banks
2. Eliminate old forms, change atomic structure
3. Balance yin-yang
4. Stimulate the hypothalamus, heal generative disease

Method

Lie down on the floor on your back. Hold the red Garnet in your palm and gaze at it for one full minute.

Place the red Garnet against the . . .

CROWN CHAKRA (top of head): Cover with palm, repeat seven times . . . "This Garnet is vibrating to open my memory banks."

SOLAR PLEXUS (near waist): Cover with palm, repeat seven times . . . "This Garnet is vibrating to balance my yin-yang."

HEART: Cover with palm, repeat seven times . . . "This Garnet is vibrating to eliminate old forms by changing the atomic structure."

RUBY

CHEMICAL COMPOSITION: $Al_2O_3(Cr)$ (Fe) (oxide ion)
CRYSTAL SYSTEM: Hexagonal (trigonal)
RED RAY
PLANET: Mars
POWER CENTER OF LOVE
HEALTH FACTOR: Strengthens the heart, blood pressure
PSYCHIC QUALITIES: Self-love, will to live

General Science

The Ruby is from the same "root" gem as the Sapphire, called "corundum," derived from the Sanskrit *kuruvinda*. The bright, clear red to pink color is caused by the element chromium replacing the aluminum of the Sapphire. Chromium causes a bright red fluorescence in the precious Ruby. A bit of ferric iron sometimes adds a slight orange cast to the red, or a slight amount of aluminum may give the red a small purplish glint.

Rubies are second in value only to Diamonds, being 9½ on the Mohs' scale of 1 to 10 in hardness. There are so few Rubies unflawed in anything over 5 carats that anything larger is more valuable than a Diamond of equal quality and size. The finest Rubies occur near Mogok, Burma, in crystals up to two inches in length. Cambodia, Thailand, Ceylon, India, Tanzania, and Australia are all sources. The latest finds have been in Norway and in the Ural Mountains of Russia. Small, pink cut Rubies are made from the pebbles gathered in streambeds of the Orient. Very few raw specimens ever leave the country of origin, as gem quality stones are immediately faceted for greater value.

History, Myth, and Magic

The name "ruby" comes from the Latin word *rubeus*, meaning the color red. In the oldest written language of the Hindus, Sanskrit, the Ruby was described as being "red as the lotus." It was also called the king of precious stones. They believed that an inextinguishable fire burned inside the gem. Modern testing has proven that it does indeed give off heat. Ruby was conferred the highest honor of being called a Brahman, the highest caste in the Hindu religion. They believed that owning a Brahman Ruby was a perfect protection against bad luck.

In Burma, where the gorgeous Ruby is their most precious commodity, they believe a Ruby must be inserted under the skin to maintain it's full protective virtues.

A Chinese writer of the thirteenth century stated that the king of Ceylon used a Ruby to rub his face daily, and he remained youthful in appearance though he lived to be ninety years of age.

There are many accountings in ancient and medieval times of Rubies glowing in the dark. In many treatises written on gems from the eleventh century through the nineteenth, almost all mention that a Ruby will grow dull when someone in the immediate family dies.

The ancient physicians equated the red stones with blood and used them in the treatment of wounds and hemorrhaging.

Healing Secrets

The Ruby does have an affect on the heart in that it is a cleansing vibration for the blood, which is the life and product of the heart.

Stress is an ever-present agent in our lives. One of its effects causes chemistry imbalance, whereby we process our food intake incorrectly, causing cholesterol to be carried in the blood instead of being disseminated. When the blood carries too much of the fatty substance, it begins to cling to the walls of the arteries and finally piles up in complete blockages. Nearly always occurring in or near the heart, these blockages cut off the flow of blood to the heart.

Anytime the circulation of blood is improved, the whole body benefits. The adrenal glands, located near the solar plexus region, are stimulated by the Ruby, which causes the heart to pump faster. Stress can also negatively affect the blood vessels of the eyes. Poor sight cannot be repaired by the Ruby (nor any other stone *at this time*), but by eliminating stress, the blood vessels in and around the eyes can function more efficiently. Their lack of constriction in turn feeds the muscles of the eyes and makes them stronger. When the muscles of the eyes are strong, vision is improved.

Psychic Strengths

The Ruby replaces the lack of self-esteem that can cause all kinds of self-destructive behavior with the vibration that teaches the holder that he is valuable and deserving of life, to the greatest heights of abundance. The Ruby will bring to its owners a sense of excitement within themselves that gives purpose to living. This is the very essence of our Creators *within* us.

The "Life Force" or "Vital Energy" resides in the sacral region and must be coaxed upward through the solar plexus to the heart. The stimulation of the solar plexus is the function of the adrenal glands, accomplished by emotional thought.

Our emotions govern every function of our bodies. The negative emotional thought that can damage our body through overstimulation of the adrenal glands is fear. The opposite of love is not hate but fear. When the Ruby is used with knowledge by the holder, fear is removed because it cannot remain in the same body with love. To truly love the self is to be rid of all guilt and fear, with the knowledge that we are capable of the same creativity and goodness as our Creator. Believing this, and affirming it while contemplating the Ruby, restores the full potential of purpose, will, and creativity to life. When these three emotions that govern the Universe are healthy in a person, they experience renewed interest in all of the facets of life, love, and passion. A belief in the positive outcome of every endeavor will then occur. Helen Keller understood and responded to this when she said, "Life is either a fantastic adventure or it is nothing."

RUBY MEDITATION

The Ruby affects the heart by providing a cleansing vibration for the blood, which, of course, is the life force and product of the heart. Anytime the circulation of the blood is improved, the whole body benefits.

The color and refraction of a Ruby is desired and needed by those whose life force requires stimulation. There is a vibration of excitement from the Ruby that gives the holder more of a zest for living.

We have known for a long time that the heart thinks on its own. When this "mind within the heart" is stimulated by wearing and meditating with a Ruby, the red ray of devotion activates a new understanding of love of self and others.

Where physical abuse can oftentimes be obvious, damage to the spirit may be almost imperceptible. It can be recognized in an individual's lack of purpose or seeming despair about continuing with life. Regular meditation with the Ruby will cause a remarkable lessening of these negative thoughts, replacing them with more positive feelings of personal security and value.

In cases where the lack of self-love has actually damaged the body or mind, the Ruby meditation needs to be used as often as possible, as many as seven times a day. It will provide emergency or rescue treatment to:

1. Increase the will toward life
2. Promote affection and acceptance of the self
3. Overcome feelings of inadequacy
4. Strengthen the heart

Method

Lie down on the floor on your back. Hold the Ruby in your palm and gaze at it for one full minute.

Place the Ruby against the . . .
SOLAR PLEXUS (near waist): Cover with palm, repeat seven times . . . "This Ruby is increasing my will toward life."
HEART: Cover with palm, repeat seven times . . . "This Ruby is vibrating to help me love myself."
FOREHEAD ("third eye"): Cover with palm, repeat seven times . . . "This Ruby is vibrating to give me self-confidence."

ROSE QUARTZ

CHEMICAL COMPOSITION: SiO_2 (silicon dioxide)
CRYSTAL SYSTEM: Hexagonal (trigonal)
SILVER and RED RAYS
PLANETS: Moon and Mars
POWER CENTER OF LOVE
HEALTH FACTORS: Mild cardiac stimulant, diuretic
PSYCHIC QUALITIES: Gentleness

General Science

The most spectacular display of Rose Quartz is in Custer, South Dakota, where there is a pink cliff almost one hundred feet long. This Rose Quartz was mined for many years and sent to China for carving. These light pink, delicate figurines are most sought after by collectors. During World War II, Rose Quartz mines were opened in Brazil, and these produce a clearer rose for carving. Brazil is the largest supplier, but the best quality comes from the Malagasy Republic (Madagascar) and Indonesia.

It is a mystery to geologists and gemologists that, unlike almost every other form of Quartz, Rose Quartz is very rarely ever found growing in crystal formations. The star or asterism often visible in Rose Quartz is seen when the gem is polished into a rounded dome shape (en cabochon).

Healing Secrets

The vibrations of the Rose Quartz act as a mild cardiac stimulant and a mild diuretic. Since water retention is a symptom of blood flow interruption, high blood pressure, and cardiac imbalance, it is convenient to treat the symptom with the cure. This is not a heavy or strong vibration stone, and it is only used for mild irregularities. Meditation encourages cheerfulness and youthfulness.

Psychic Strengths

The light passing through the Rose Quartz is rotating the plane of polarization in the pyramidal formation. The effect on the mental level is to decrease the willful assertiveness of conquest in personal relationships or career. The polarity of the yin-yang must be rotated with a softening of the love intensity. The muscular love of force must be polarized into the naive, innocent love of a young child, who gives with no thought of reciprocity. A general softening of the attitude first toward the self and then toward others who are seen as restrictors will be encouraged by meditation with Rose Quartz.

The pink rays, working through the Rose Quartz in the

heart area, soften the demanding Mars vibrations with the receptiveness of the Moon's rays.

ROSE QUARTZ MEDITATION

Rose Quartz is not a heavy or strong vibrational stone and is only used for mild irregularities.

Meditation with Rose Quartz will effect a general softening of the "me first" attitude while it also encourages cheerfulness and youthfulness. Among its attributes it:

1. Promotes return to innocent love
2. Softens the attitude toward self-restrictions
3. Rotates polarity for balance
4. Acts as mild cardiac stimulant and diuretic

Method

Lie down on the floor on your back. Hold the Rose Quartz in your palm and gaze at it for one full minute.

Place the Rose Quartz against the . . .

SOLAR PLEXUS (near waist): Cover with palm, repeat seven times . . . "This Rose Quartz is vibrating to help me return to the innocent love I knew as a child."

HEART: Cover with palm, repeat seven times . . . "This Rose Quartz is vibrating to help me be more gentle and easy with myself."

FOREHEAD ("third eye"): Cover with palm, repeat seven times . . . "This Rose Quartz is vibrating to keep my polarities in rotation."

Saturn
The Green Ray

CHRYSOPRASE ◆ EMERALD ◆ JADE ◆ MALACHITE ◆

PERIDOT ◆ GREEN GARNET

"The human body is made up of electronic vibrations. Each *organ* and organism has its electronic unit of vibration necessary for the sustenance of, and equilibrium in, that particular organism. A low electrical charge may be set up by the vibratory impulse of certain gems and minerals that can be transferred to the body, causing it to extract more of the particular element in digested foods."

—**Edgar Cayce**
The New York Times
Oct. 9, 1910

▲▲▲

Saturn's cosmic vibrations, traveling on the green ray, enter our body in the "mind power center area of order" near the solar plexus. This physical mind center of order, located behind the navel, has been understood by meta-

140

physicians for centuries. The ancient Greek philosopher Philolaos wrote about the solar plexus. Madame Blavatsky, founder of Theosophy, believed this theory of the center of order, as did Edgar Cayce, the most famous American psychic and diagnostic healer of our time.

The common slang expression that pinpoints specifically this area proves that even the least educated among us can depend on that "mind center" to tell the truth when we say we have a "gut feeling" about something.

Saturn is the teacher who gives to us a stern command that we must have order in our daily lives, and who keeps us on course. Saturn's rays cause us to have conflict and inner struggle because our animal, earthly nature often causes us to desire actions that are in direct opposition to our spiritual evolution.

On the purely physical plane, the disruption of our home life, and an inability to function efficiently in our work, are directly related to a lack of physical order. This can be expressed as untidyness, clutter, or laziness. The accumulation of useless materials and the scattering of objects is in direct opposition to the universal law of order. It is a physical form of mental disorder. Eventually this lack of order will express itself in physical illness.

On the mental plane, when thought is not consistently directed or focused, the mind may become easily distracted. Often desires may never be fulfilled because lack of direction makes beginning impossible. It is very common to hear this expressed by people who are dissatisfied with their present situation and say they want to make a change but don't know what to do or where to begin. It takes willpower to establish order.

In our emotional world, the lack of harmony may be so imperceptible that one may give the appearance of order. Yet even though the mental and physical aspects may be in evidence, a subtle emotional imbalance may occur. The first emotional indiscretion is protection of self through excuses or a belief in that which is untruth. Saturn is the planet of truth. It has been said that if all judgment were left to Saturn, we would receive justice without mercy.

To guarantee the proper balance of mental, physical, and emotional order, this solar plexus center of thinking must be trained. Here is the seat of emotion, the home of the little child in each of us. Saturn is a strict teacher. If we allow our impatient emotions to go unbridled, Saturn is always there to place restrictions upon the outcome of our impatient actions.

One major aspect of life's purpose is to discover and appreciate our individual value and ability. We choose families into which we are born who will either aid or restrict us according to the strength we need to acquire in the exercise. Very few children escape the trauma of some kind of family dynamic that causes humiliation or anger to breed. The lesson that finally strengthens and evolves the soul is the struggle to take responsibility for our own destiny. Karmic retribution inherent in Saturn assures that whatever we do to someone will be done to us in return, whether positive or negative.

The basic movement of all living, growing, evolving things is upward and forward toward the light. To "come clean" with the truth is to see that we chose that very situation as a test of our ability to evolve against obstacles. The drive of the subconscious in our lives is to make us happy, so it always tells the truth.

Accepting the Divine order of all things and adjusting our attitude against disharmony will relieve us from a most tiring responsibility, that of value judgment. Our own so-called mistakes, as well as those of others, can be seen as they are, a part of the necessary pattern to growth and life.

Maturity is the sign of Saturn. Maturity and wisdom are the criteria for evolution, the results of self-mastery, and provide the courage to deal with reality. Self-esteem cannot be dependent upon the values of others. When we can accept responsibility for our own decisions and the consequences of our choices, we begin to detect the guiding hand of our strict but perfect teacher.

The green ray of active intelligence is the color chosen for the currency of the United States; it is symbolic to our national financial success. Saturn rules the tenth house of the Zodiac, called the house of "status," or of station in life and career. This is most often linked to money as the physical, material reward for a job well done.

CHRYSOPRASE

(Quartz family, chalcedony group)
CHEMICAL COMPOSITION: SiO_2 (silicon dioxide)
CRYSTAL SYSTEM: Hexagonal (trigonal)
GREEN RAY
PLANET: Saturn
POWER CENTERS OF WILL AND POWER
HEALTH FACTORS: Thyroid and diet control
PSYCHIC QUALITIES: Addictions, overindulgence

General Science

Chrysoprase is a translucent, opaque, apple-green member of the Quartz group of semiprecious stones. It has several cousins: Aventurine (also green but with mica sparkles), Rose Quartz, Tiger's-eye, Cat's-eye, Hawk's-eye, Cornelian Heliotrope, and Agates. It has a hardness of 6½–7 on the Mohs' scale. It is the most valuable of all the chalcedony group because it is the most rare.

It is found as nodules, resembling petrified gel, in nickel ore deposits. It first found favor in Poland around the 1300s when it was discovered in the area of Frankenstein. That mine is now worked out. Around 1960, a good quality was discovered in Queensland, Australia. It is also found in Brazil, India, the Malagasy Republic, South Africa, the Russian Urals, and the United States in Arizona, California, and Oregon.

History, Myth, and Magic

In earlier times Chrysoprase was used in much the same manner as Lapis Lazuli, for interior decoration. Some beautiful examples are the Wenceslous Chapel in Prague, and Sanssouci Castle near Berlin.

Chrysoprase has been found in the jewelry of Egyptian mummies. There is a very special necklace of amulets in the Egyptian collection of the Berlin Museum, dating back to 1500 B.C.

Steinbuch Volmar, writing in 1877, related ancient powers of the Chrysoprase to the miraculous protection from execution, by holding a piece in the mouth!

Healing Secrets

Julia Lorusso and Joel Glick in their book *Healing Stones* (Brotherhood of Life, Albuquerque, NM, 1976) give the Chrysoprase a very high rating in its present state of evolution. The information they have received through channeling from Universal Intelligence relates the vibration of the Chrysoprase to two specific physical areas of the body. These two higher chakras, the throat and crown chakras, are protected by the Chrysoprase.

The light frequency emitted by the gem is taken into

the body through the optic nerve into the glands of the brain. In Eastern philosophy this portion of the body physical is related to a metaphysical point of power, called the crown chakra. The crown of the head represents the physical portion of the body, where the vibrations from certain planets in our galaxy enter the body. The glands in the brain activated by the Chrysoprase effect the distribution of chemicals derived from food.

The thyroid and parathyroid systems near the throat chakra, and the pineal and pituitary ductless glands near the crown chakra, regulate the total distribution of the body chemicals. If there is any deviation from the highest and best state of the dense body of the individual, the Chrysoprase will protect these glands and regulate distribution.

Psychic Strengths

The Chrysoprase has a mutable vibration that can adapt to the vibration of the wearer. Like a chameleon, it adjusts itself as a screening device allowing only things of the highest nature to pass through the throat and crown chakras of the wearer. It measures each vibration of every word, sound, idea, or emotion that seeks to invade the consciousness of the wearer. Only those vibrations that match the inherent higher vibration of the individual are allowed to pass through. It can be compared to a modern technological "voice print" identifier.

If the individual has been susceptible to being swept up into the negative life problems of friends, relatives, and acquaintances, the Chrysoprase will screen out and deflect these vibrations. This is not to say the person will become callous or unsympathetic to others. It will provide a shield against overinvolvement. In turn the mind will be protected from distraction, and it will see the truth that each individual "sets up" their own lessons, builds their own karma, and must truly live through and experience each portion to grow.

CHRYSOPRASE MEDITATION

Chrysoprase affects the throat and crown chakras, shielding the thyroid and pituitary glandular systems in those areas.

Chrysoprase will aid in regulating any type of overindulgence of the body or imagination and will restrict unhealthy impulses. Worn at the throat or as earrings, it will have a much quicker and more directed effect on these areas as well as on the entire body to:

1. Shield the thyroid and pituitary glands
2. Screen against harmful substances passing through the mouth and head
3. Literally and figuratively clear the vision
4. Mentally and physically restrict overexpansion

Whether or not one is attracted to this stone on sight is not important. If it is suggested for regulation of body chemical distribution or for control of overindulgence, it will make a friend of itself.

If the gem is worn constantly and handled often, there will be a bonded affinity. Its chameleon quality to blend vibrations will truly arouse a sympathetic vibration in the wearer.

Method

Lie down on the floor on your back. Hold the Chrysoprase in your palm and gaze at it for one full minute.

Place the Chrysoprase against the . . .

SOLAR PLEXUS (near waist): Cover with palm, repeat seven times . . . "This Chrysoprase is vibrating to screen all substances entering my body."

HEART: Cover with palm, repeat seven times . . . "This Chrysoprase is vibrating to shield me from overexpansion."

FOREHEAD ("third eye"): Cover with palm, repeat seven times . . . "This Chrysoprase is vibrating to clear my vision."

EMERALD

(Cyclosilicate group, beryl, silicate)

CHEMICAL COMPOSITION: $Be_3Al_2(Si_6O_{18})$

CRYSTAL SYSTEM: Hexagonal in prism and pinacoid forms

GREEN RAY

PLANET: Saturn

POWER CENTER OF ORDER

HEALTH FACTORS: Skeleton, bones, spine

PSYCHIC QUALITIES: Honesty, love to others, self-disclosure

General Science

In ancient Greek the term *beryllos* signified a green stone. Today, beryl is used to identify a certain crystal system.

The Emerald belongs to this structural system, as do the Aquamarines, Morganite, and Goshenite. Differences occur in these stones because of the specific elements within the structure, which give them individual colors and special vibrations.

The element that gives the Emerald its specific clear green color is chromium. Emeralds commonly have inclusions of milky white streaks or clouds. Naturally the clearer an Emerald is, the greater is its value. On a scale of 1 to 10, it measures 8 in hardness. It differs from other precious stones because it remains the same color in both natural and artificial lighting. The non-gem varieties are used as a source of the light metal, beryllium.

The most outstanding deposits are found in Colombia and Brazil. Emerald mines are located in many regions, including Russia, Austria, Africa, India, Pakistan, Ontario in Canada, and North Carolina in the United States.

History, Myth, and Magic

The Roman Emperor Nero had a magnificent Emerald through which he viewed the gladiators. Cleopatra, Queen of Egypt, wore wonderful Emeralds from her own mine in upper Egypt. The Egyptians are often linked to the Incas and Mayas of South America because both cultures were able to construct huge pyramids without modern machinery. The Colombian Emerald mines are among the world's richest. The Egyptians and Incas share these two things in common. Are Emeralds responsible in any way for the mental abilities of the two cultures? Or could both cultures have originated on a now sunken continent where the use of gems was employed and understood by a culture much more advanced than our present one? Do the Emeralds have any relationship to the pyramids?

There is gem lore from biblical times that attributes the

vibration of kindness to the Emerald. Medieval understanding of the Emerald was that its vibrations held the key to success in love. Magicians of that day were also aware that the Emerald had a special influence. Their tricks and potions would not develop correctly unless an Emerald was present. If they were false or deceitful in their alchemy, the Emerald would cause them to fail. This is another evolutionary link that still corroborates the original properties of the Emerald: honesty, intuition, and love.

A talismanic Emerald of a rich, deep green and weighing 78 carats was once the property of the Mogul emperors of Delhi. Engraved around the outer edges in Persian script were the words, "The special protection of God is with this charm."

Healing Secrets

The therapeutic use of gemstones can be traced back to the ancient histories of both India and Egypt. The Ebers Papyrus, an uncovered Egyptian treasure, gives many prescriptions for using gems. The next historical source is *The Natural History of Pliny* (Gaius Plinius: A.D. 23–79). It carries forth all the ancient accounts of gem therapy known at that time.

The Greek historian Theophrastus wrote a detailed description of the effect of Emerald on the eyes around 300 B.C. When Paracelsus (1493–1541) began exploring the actual elements in gems, he wrote that the Emerald contained copper. He was mistaken about copper—we know it is chromium—but he was one of the pioneers in equating the elements in gems to the elements in human bodies.

Century after century writings are studied and compiled and many times are rewritten by new authorities. New discoveries of ancient evidence have been added, and old documents have been retranslated. But the predominant theme is some unknown emanation of subtle power from the stone itself that will cure an affected area of the body when held or worn against it.

The Emerald is one of the most powerful healing stones. It demands a complete honesty and the giving out of love from the healer. Because Saturn rules the skeleton, bones, and teeth, it is most effective in these areas, as well as the internal areas behind the navel in the "order" center. The spinal bony structure is most often the target of pain when life is out of order. Emeralds held on these areas can be a relief. Healing occurs when order is restored. Broken bones or teeth can be temporarily anesthetized by using the Emerald as a transmitter for Saturn's ray-waves. It will also promote new structure or knitting of breaks.

Refusal to "see" the truth causes eye problems. The eyes can also be strengthened by meditation with the Emerald.

Deterioration of eyesight is often linked with sugar diabetes. This crippling disease of imbalance within the chemical system can often be traced back to "the mind power center of order," the area of the pancreas. Coming clean with the truth, resetting priorities, changing one's attitude toward money or financial security, can often bring relief. Meditation with the Emerald can speed up this "eye opening" and relieve symptoms. Understanding brings inner order. Inner order brings health.

Psychic Strengths

Throughout the tracing threads of history, the vibration of the Emerald has been a message concerning Truth (honesty) and Love (giving, receiving, and understanding). There are several diseases that affect the human body if these two vibrations are weak.

For instance, if we refuse to "see" the truth, our eyesight

will be affected. If we only think about getting or receiving love, creating a greediness for sweetness, we may be more likely to contract sugar diabetes. If we do not give out love to another person, then we give it to something. The substitute is often money. If we grasp for it, we may panic, and panic causes muscles to tighten, creating pain in the back and neck. We may love the thing that takes away that pain of fear—total involvement in a job or our own body. These misplaced loves cause all manner of poisons to pour into our digestive tract.

EMERALD MEDITATION

The Emerald is one of the most powerful healing stones, demanding complete honesty and love from the healer.

The spinal bony structure is often the target of pain when life is out of order. An Emerald held on these areas can bring relief. Healing occurs when order is restored.

When truth is explored and acceptance of personal choices is made, the love withheld inside can pour out. As soon as we begin to give out love, we begin to receive it.

Meditation with the Emerald speeds up the "eye opening" process and will:

1. Expose subconscious belief systems
2. Clear the conscience
3. Force love OUT from the holder
4. Strengthen the back and spine

Method

Lie down on the floor on your back. Hold the Emerald in your palm and gaze at it for one full minute.

Place the Emerald against the . . .
SOLAR PLEXUS (near waist): Cover with palm, repeat seven times . . . "This Emerald is vibrating to help me 'come clean' with the truth."
HEART: Cover with palm, repeat seven times . . . "This Emerald is vibrating to help me give out love."
FOREHEAD ("third eye"): Cover with palm, repeat seven times . . . "This Emerald is vibrating so I may know myself as I truly am, a loving, giving, trusting person."

JADE-JADEITE

CHEMICAL COMPOSITION: Inosilicate $NaAl(Si_2O_6)$ (sodium aluminum silicate)
CRYSTAL SYSTEM: Monoclinic, very rare to see actual crystals
GREEN RAY
PLANET: Saturn
POWER CENTER OF ORDER
HEALTH FACTOR: Knees, skeleton, gall bladder, duodenum
PSYCHIC QUALITIES: Problem identification, problem solving

General Science

There are several colors of Jade, from a very dark, opaque green to a slightly translucent pink through white. The other colors are rust, lilac, and black. There are two types of Jade, called Jadeite and Nephrite. The most valuable are colored by chromium to an intense emerald green called Jadeite. It is harder than Nephrite and can be tested by scraping it with a knife because it will not scratch. The pure green Jadeite is often called Imperial Jade, the very best deposits of which, found in Burma, are used for carving. The natives in Burma can walk in the streams and feel the Jade with their bare feet.

Jade is formed in long needles, or felted masses of tiny, interlocked crystals, so it is extremely tough. On the Mohs' scale of 1 to 10, it is 6½–7 in hardness. It is fairly easy to carve, but difficult to split.

Nephrite-Jade is found in the U.S. in Wyoming and Alaska. It is also found in New Zealand, Germany, Siberia, and China.

History, Myth, and Magic

Some of the oldest finds of Jade artifacts are ax heads, dating back to prehistoric cave people. There have been finds of this kind in Europe, Asia, and Mexico. For many years there was speculation about whether Jade artifacts found in Mexico indicated that this continent was either settled by or had traded with Asians. If there were Jade mines in Mexico, they have been lost.

When the Spanish came to conquer the Aztecs, they found Jade used as talismans and weapons. One of the Aztec gods of fire, Xuihtecutli, presided over the ear-piercing ceremony of young boys and girls. His shield had five large jade pieces set in gold in the form of a cross. The Aztecs called Jade the hip stone because it was worn over the kidney as a cure for disease. The Spanish translation of this name was *piedra de hijade* from *hijada*. The English mutation is "Jade."

Jade carvings worn as ornament are very ancient in the symbolism of the Orient. A carved Jade phoenix is bestowed upon young girls when they come of age. The gift to a newlywed couple of a carving in Jade of a unicorn and a butterfly signifies success in romance, and so is often given to one's fiancée.

The Chinese share a custom that has also been discovered by archaeologists in Egyptian, Mayan, and North American Indian cultures, which is putting a stone in the mouth of the dead before burial.

The Chinese were said to love the music of the Jade. They made instruments like wind chimes or carved pendants that could be struck for their melodious ring. This stone chime was reported to have been a tranquilizer for the famous moralist, reformer K'ung–Fu-Tse (551–479 B.C.), whom we know as Confucius.

In practically every museum of any note all over the world, a collection of Jade carvings can be found. This high art form is admired by every culture. In the Museum of Natural History in New York is a New Zealand Jade belonging to the Maori that weighs seven thousand pounds. This is the largest mass of Jade ever found.

Healing Secrets

There is a correspondence between the physical areas and the metaphysical areas activated by the Jade. The "third eye," or knowing part of the brain, is activated more than is necessary in some individuals. When their emotional vibrations are weaker than their intellect, it alters the production of bile by the liver and causes it to change in consistency and color. The bile is found in the gall bladder and is discharged into the duodenum to help in digestion, especially of fats. The Jade has a vibration that will balance the amount of emotion to the amount of intellect. This would result in the bile being distributed evenly and perfectly into the system. This insures a healthy gall bladder and duodenum.

If the opposite condition exists and a person exhibits an imbalance of exaggerated emotions along with conditioned intellectual response, this softens the muscles supporting the colon, kidneys, and liver. This condition may manifest itself in various ailments of those areas, allowing these organs to sag and press against each other and resulting in a displacement. The blood vessels also lack support in the lower area and may stretch and balloon into hemorrhoids or other varicose veins. The Jade has the vibration to bring tension back into the muscles surrounding these areas into a perfect polarity and balanced comfort. When this is accomplished through meditation with the Jade, tenseness of the colon and constipation will be relieved. The balanced chemical content of the bile will promote a healthy liver, gall bladder, and stomach.

Psychic Strengths

Jade acts as a stimulant to the Emotional Body, penetrating into body-remembered feelings that have been felt in many lifetimes. The Jade stimulates the emotional memory to discover karma (lessons we must learn in this lifetime in order to evolve) so that we can uncover past-life remembrances. Modern psychology has worked for years on the assumption that our personal relationships with the opposite sex are almost totally dependent on our relationship with the parent during infancy. This does not take into account habits or mind-sets included in our current state of reincarnated evolution. We may be here on Earth at this time to "work out" or learn to understand the perfect way to relate to others. When we meditate with a Jade, we penetrate into these emotions and discover where we may have missed our mark in the past. If we realize that we made certain decisions in another lifetime, we are relieved of the tension buildup inside of us caused by condemning ourselves for mistakes in our present life. In this way, we can cease to carry around dead weight from the past and can progress into our present and future.

The Jade vibration has a psychic effect on the heart, the point in the psyche where the intellect meets the emotions. In the actual physical body it is halfway between the brain and the solar plexus. The Egyptian civilization put particular emphasis on the heart. Theologians, philosophers, and scientists have for centuries wondered, where does a soul live in the body? Many ancients have believed it to be in the heart.

JADE MEDITATION

Jade acts as a stimulant to the emotions to penetrate our body's memory, where feelings may have had inappropriate reactions for several lifetimes. Jade helps us discover lessons we must learn in this lifetime (karma) in order to evolve.

The vibration of Jade can uncover past-life remembrances. Through meditation, Jade can penetrate these emotions, pinpointing where we may have missed our mark in the past.

Jade also has a psychic effect on the heart at the point where the intellect meets the emotions. If the heart accepts too much emotion and turns away the mind, it becomes like quicksand, too soft to stand on. On the other hand, if emotion finds no admittance, the heart becomes a hard place where nothing is comfortable.

Meditation with Jade produces a balance of emotion and intellect. Added together the sum total is wisdom. In modern semantics we would call this "someone who is all heart."

In addition to stimulating our total being to penetrate the camouflage surrounding a problem, Jade will:

1. Stimulate a solution
2. Balance intellect with emotion
3. Clear the liver, kidneys, and duodenum

Method

Lie down on the floor on your back. Hold the Jade in your palm and gaze at it for one full minute.

Place the Jade against the . . .

SOLAR PLEXUS (near waist): Cover with palm, repeat seven times . . . "This Jade is vibrating to balance my emotions and my intellect."

HEART: Cover with palm, repeat seven times . . . "This Jade is vibrating to raise my desire to know the truth."

FOREHEAD ("third eye"): Cover with palm, repeat seven times . . . "This Jade is vibrating to help me penetrate the problem and solve it."

MALACHITE

CHEMICAL COMPOSITION: $Cu_2Co_3(OH)_2$ (basic copper carbonate)
CRYSTAL SYSTEM: Monoclinic
GREEN RAY
PLANET: Saturn
POWER CENTER OF ORDER
HEALTH FACTORS: Teeth, jaw
PSYCHIC QUALITIES: Patience, self-control

General Science

The early Greek writers Theophrastus and Pliny called this green-circled stone "false emerald." The Greek word for a group of plants including okra and marshmallow is *malache*, and their word for soft, *malakos*, may have been combined to describe this very soft, green mineral originally spelled "Molochites."

The softness of the stone (it measures only 4 on the Mohs' scale) makes it easy to carve into figurines. It does not seem to inhibit its use as jewelry, and it is very popular smoothly polished, en cabochon, in pendants, rings, bracelets, etc.

Crystals are very rare, but specimens and stalactites that resemble bubbles or bunches of grapes are popular collectors' items. When sliced and polished, the alternating light- and dark-green circles are captivating. The polishing of spheres or egg shapes have been popular in all ages.

Malachite is sensitive to heat (hot water) and acids (ammonia), so do not wear jewelry while washing dishes, cleaning, or in the Jacuzzi.

Russia had the most important finds of Malachite from

the Ural Mountains during the time of the czars. They used much of it in the interior decoration of their palaces.

Zaire, in Central Africa, now produces the highest quality and quantity. Deposits are also found in Arizona in the United States, as well as in Australia, Chile, Zimbabwe, and South Africa.

History, Myth, and Magic

Malachite mines were worked between the Suez Canal and the Sinai desert as early as 4000 B.C. The mines of King Solomon produced copper and Malachite.

The ground powder of Malachite was used by all women of that early age, in the areas supplied by the mines, as a beauty aid in the form of eye shadow.

The ground Malachite has also been used for centuries to produce color for painting leaves and foliage—as Lapis Lazuli was used for blue.

In the Egyptian collection of the Berlin Museum are many pieces of jewelry dating back to 1500 B.C. Taken from tombs and mummies of wealthy Egyptians, many bracelets and necklaces are found to contain Malachite beads and carved figures or amulets.

The Malachite, polished to show its circles, was called peacock stone as it resembled the eye in a peacock feather. The gem was usually triangular, mounted in silver, and worn as an amulet against the "evil eye."

Healing Secrets

With Malachite's being one of the several gems that receive the green ray from Saturn, the emphasis is on the hard structures of the body. Emerald affects the spine; Jade affects the skeleton; Malachite affects the teeth.

All abscesses, cavities, and diseases concerning the teeth

and bones surrounding the teeth can be improved by using the Malachite in meditation and wearing it on the body. Wearing it as close as possible to the jaw is preferable.

The recent discovery of a jaw displacement problem, medically called tempero mandibular jaw (when the lower jawbone is not in line with the upper), has brought attention to the effect of stress on the teeth. The muscles in the neck constrict to such a degree that the lower jaw is pulled out of alignment. This causes the bite to be off center, which in turn causes an equal reaction of other facial muscles to compensate for chewing inefficiency. The teeth begin to shift and relocate in an effort to realign. Headaches and finally even stomach problems can develop through this obscure reaction to stress.

Saturn's influence through cosmic rays is in dealing with stress. It is also concerned with structure—both in the physical and metaphysical areas of life on Earth. In order to build any structure, there must be a proper amount of stress for it to be substantial. Any architect, carpenter, or engineer is aware of this principle. Too much stress on any construction, building, or body will cause its collapse. The grinding or gritting of the teeth is a physical manifestation of an improper reaction to the stress caused by impatience. There is a definite correlation of the impatience of the individual to restrictions imposed by Saturn. In the psyche of the sufferer, the natural working of joints (including the jaw) is restricted and begins to cause a malfunction on a physical level. Using the Malachite as an aid to acquiring patience through meditation will relieve many problems of the jawbone and teeth.

Psychic Strengths

The psychic properties of Malachite are focused on building structure into the foundation of the life. There are natural Universal Laws that are constantly in operation all around and within us. We speak of building our lives just as we speak of building a bridge. We all have instinctual knowledge of the laws of structure, visible to us in the world and cosmos around us. We build our physical bodies through the laws of exercise and diet—just as we build our character through right action and right thinking. The psychic qualities of Malachite are the restrictions that guide us to structure our minds and bodies toward patience with our own growth and the actions of those around us.

MALACHITE MEDITATION

All abscesses, cavities, and disease concerning the teeth and the bones surrounding the teeth can be improved by using the Malachite in meditation and wearing it on the body, preferably as close to the jaw as possible.

The grinding and gritting of teeth is a physical manifestation of an improper reaction to the stress caused by impatience. Using the Malachite will aid in acquiring patience and will relieve many problems of the jawbone and teeth.

Saturn's cosmic vibrations, traveling on the green ray, enter our body in the "mind power area of order." This center of thinking must be trained to guarantee the proper balance of stress because order is the first law of structure.

Wearing Malachite and using it as an aid in daily active meditation will give our lives proper structure, order, and the patience to right action and reaction. You will find:

1. Increased patience toward self and situations
2. Order and structure will begin to manifest themselves in life
3. Healthier teeth and jaws

Method

Lie down on the floor on your back. Hold the Malachite in your palm and gaze at it for one full minute.

Place the Malachite against the . . .

SOLAR PLEXUS (near waist): Cover with palm, repeat seven times . . . "This Malachite is vibrating to increase patience with myself and situations."

HEART: Cover with palm, repeat seven times . . . "This Malachite is vibrating to help me use the proper amount of stress."

FOREHEAD ("third eye"): Cover with palm, repeat seven times . . . "This Malachite is vibrating to help me bring order into the structure of my life."

PERIDOT

(Neosilicate Group)
CHEMICAL COMPOSITION: Fe_2SiO_4 (fayalite)
CRYSTAL SYSTEM: Orthorhombic
YELLOW and GREEN RAYS
PLANET: Jupiter and Saturn
POWER CENTER OF ELIMINATION
HEALTH FACTOR: Lower back, strength, elimination
PSYCHIC QUALITIES: Spiritual increasing

General Science

The color of this clear transparent gem, whose mineralogical names have been varied, is yellow/olive-green. George F. Kunz, a leading American mineralogist of the 1900s, referred to Peridot as Chrysolite. Contemporary mineralogist John Sinkankas called Peridot by the name Olivine. The German naturalist Johann Forster called the brownish variety Forsterite, after himself. The true yellow-green variety is called Fayalite because it was found on the island of Fayal in the Azores. The word *Peridot* is derived from middle French and is the common English title for this precious yellow-green stone. Even *Webster's* does not give the origin of its meaning. On a hardness scale of 1 to 10, it measures 6½.

The Peridot has a significant double light refraction that helps to differentiate it from several other gems, such as Golden Beryl, Chrysoberyl, demantoid green Garnet, synthetic Spinel, Emerald, or Tourmaline.

The most important Peridot mines are located on the Island of St. John, in the Red Sea, 188 miles from Aswan, Egypt. It is a volcanic island typical of other known deposits of Peridot. The mine has been operating for 3,500 years. Other quarries are located in Mogok (Burma), Australia, Brazil, South Africa, Zaire, Norway, and in the United States, Arizona, Hawaii, and New Mexico. The largest cut Peridot (310 carats) is part of the Smithsonian Collection in Washington, D.C., and was mined in St. John.

History, Myth, and Magic

The most ancient reference to Peridot appeared around 5000 B.C. in the Hebrew Old Testament. The stone is listed as the second gem on the breastplate of the high priest (Exodus 28:15–30). There has been considerable confusion concerning the name of the second stone, especially because of the many names used for the gem we now call Peridot. However, most research has determined that the gem was indeed Peridot, which would have been available in the nearby locality of Aswan, Egypt, and also soft enough to be easily inscribed. The stone on the breastplate bears the name of the tribe "Simeon" on its surface.

When the Crusaders returned to Europe from their religious exploits, they brought gems—including Peridot. This was its first introduction into Europe and may have been when its French name was first used. At about the same time, writings of Arabic origin were circulated in Europe, including a "Dream Book," attributed to the author Achametis. In dreams, Peridot had two meanings, one signifying faith and religious devotion to God, the other reminding the dreamer to observe caution.

Peridots from the Crusades eventually found their way into cathedral treasures in Europe. The most notable are in the Treasury of the Three Magi, in the Dome at Cologne, West Germany. Some of these Peridots measure two inches long.

During the Baroque period (1550–1750), the Peridot was much favored. It was included in many designs as Europeans embellished everything with gold, gilt, ruffles, scrolls, and jewels.

The Baroque period was so extremely overbalanced in wasteful decoration and the spending of public funds for purely aesthetic sensibilities that it became grotesque. The impoverished masses were incensed, and the French Revolution was born. The monied class worked with the vibrations of the Peridot to the extent they set themselves up vainly as perfect models of aesthetic culture. This so outraged the masses that it brought about a totally new age of understanding. Every revolution begins with an extreme.

Peridot is a gem born out of two spectacular birthplaces. The most well-known is the volcano; the most unusual is the meteor. One kind of stony iron meteorite called pallasite has Peridot crystals embedded in it like chocolate chips. There are cut gems from meteorites! How exciting to own a heaven-sent jewel, and how appropriate that it should be part of something from outside our world as well as from deep inside.

The most prominent volcanic Peridots are found at the Kojo volcano near Honolulu, Hawaii. In Arizona, the Peridot is mined for us by the ants. In making their many-layered dwellings, ants run into Peridot pebbles. To finish their architecture as planned, they push the pebbles up and out into a waste pile, making a most attractive—and valuable—ant hill. Anyone can pick them up. Long necklaces of these pebbles were strung and worn by American Indians in the Southwest and by Polynesian natives for many centuries.

Healing Secrets

The Peridot corresponds to the Sun. The Sun corresponds to the center of our body, the solar plexus. This is the area of our body that is the balanced center of gravity and of space. It is a network of nerves containing ganglia that send nerve impulses to the abdominal viscera. Ganglia are centers of force, energy, and activity. In plain language, they form the other brain . . . the part of ourselves that responds or corresponds to the most basic center of the Universe. In this area we experience the heights and depths of emotion. We experience extreme fear, total disappointment, sexual excitement, and spiritual ecstasy.

Since the Peridot's vibration corresponds to this area, it can decipher messages from the solar plexus for us. It can identify the necessary and weed out the unnecessary. In this way, it is particularly soothing to the digestion and stomach, and will regulate adrenaline. All diseases of the elimination systems and abdominal diseases are improved by meditation with and by wearing the Peridot.

Psychic Strengths

As the Peridot itself comes from the depths of the Earth through volcanoes and from outer space in meteorites, it corresponds to the limits of human emotion. This gem has a double refraction, meaning it takes light (understanding) and sends it in two directions. Its vibrations go directly to the solar plexus and to the other brain. It promotes an opening of good communication between those two centers.

When these centers are in balance, the result is that each reaches out to the other with a meeting in the middle of the heart. When this happens, the soul is truly born, and spiritual light comes.

Light has always been the symbol for understanding. The Sun of our galaxy provides our daylight. The Moon of our Earth provides our night light by reflection from the Sun. Everything that we observe in our outer existence is also true of our inner life. Everything small corresponds to something large . . . large-to-small, inner-to-outer.

In our historical symbology, the Sun has always represented the male thrust or activator. The Moon represents the softer female receiver. Both are light, and both are influential to certain workings of the elements on Earth. Both reign at their proper time. They correspond to our brain (the Sun) and our solar plexus (the Moon). The Sun shines in great bursts of activity, striking out and sending its energy to us. The Moon glows, gently but firmly, and changes the amount of reflection given back—seemingly by its own will.

The Peridot contains a vibrational correspondence to action and control, to Sun and Moon, to heart and head, to inner Earth and outer space, to the spirit within a human and the great spirit of the Universe. The light of understanding in every major spiritual quest finally must reconcile these things as they appear to be so opposite and separate from each other. The Peridot has a gentle vibration—to calm the whirling contradictions, to slow down the solar plexus, slow down the other brain, and put them in rhythmic balance.

The Peridot is an arbitrator or a moderator. It acts as a liaison between emotion and reason. The life-force energy is the spark that activates the mass of neutrons, protons, electrons, etc. that cling together and vibrate in different rhythms to create the illusion of human life. So far, as we have yet discovered, only one vibration on our Earth plane has a third element. The human vibration contains a form of light that we call understanding. All the rest have energy and mass. In the beginning, it is written that the Creators said, "Let there be light." This light—understanding—the third element, is the soul. The Peridot is to be worn and used by awakened persons who truly desire to know their own soul.

PERIDOT MEDITATION

The Peridot corresponds to the center of our body, the solar plexus. This area of our body is the balanced center of gravity and of space. Of this area we can say, "I feel it in my guts," for it is here that we experience the heights and depths of emotion.

The messages received by the solar plexus go directly to the stomach and heart, where they must be monitored to adjust the chemicals released into the body for fight-or-flight action.

Peridot deciphers these messages, identifying and eliminating what is either necessary or unnecessary. Because it regulates release of adrenaline, it is particularly soothing to the digestion.

It acts as an arbitrator and moderator, providing the liaison between emotion and reason.

The Peridot is to be worn and used by persons who truly desire to know their own soul. Meditation with this gem will:

1. Increase spiritual awareness
2. Eliminate psychological blocks and negative beliefs
3. Refresh the spirit body
4. Soothe the solar plexus and elimination tracts

Method

Lie down on the floor on your back. Hold the Peridot in your palm and gaze at it for one full minute.

Place the Peridot against the . . .

SOLAR PLEXUS (near waist): Cover with palm, repeat seven times . . . "This Peridot is vibrating to increase my spiritual awareness."

HEART: Cover with palm, repeat seven times . . . "This Peridot is vibrating to eliminate negative beliefs."

FOREHEAD: ("third eye"): Cover with palm, repeat seven times . . . "This Peridot is vibrating to eliminate prejudice against my spiritual growth."

GREEN GARNET

(Andradite)
CHEMICAL COMPOSITION: $Ca_3Fe_2(SiO_4)_3$
CRYSTAL SYSTEM: Isometric
GREEN RAY
PLANET: Saturn
POWER CENTER OF ORDER
HEALTH FACTOR: Back and spine, deposits in joints, spastic colon
PSYCHIC QUALITIES: Reestablish order, relief from pressure

General Science

Green Garnet, also called Andradite, was named after Portuguese mineralogist, J. B. Andrada (1765–1838). The most recognized color is an almost emerald green, sometimes with yellow or brown casts. It measures 6½ on a hardness scale of 1 to 10. Gem quality stones are mined near Vesuvius and in the Alban Hills near Rome, Italy. The most beautiful of all are found in Russia in the Ural Mountains.

Healing Secrets

If the Andradite Garnet can be used for seven minutes in meditation every day and worn as jewelry with the full understanding of its properties, it will improve problems affecting the back and spine, deposits in the joints, and spastic colon, all of which are directly caused by incorrect mind-set.

The wine-red Garnet transmits from planet Pluto, but the Green Garnet is under the influence of Saturn. Saturn is described by astrologers as "the teacher." It sends impulses that will stop us in the process of any situation unless we are working from right motive. Saturn is a restrictor, a constrictor, a disciplinarian.

The Green Garnet is finding favor among those who feel the quality of the Emeralds being mined now is not exactly clear. Since Green Garnet is not known to grow in large crystals, however, it is somewhat rare and slightly less valuable than the Emerald.

Psychic Strengths

The Green Garnet is vibrating at a rate of change. It helps us to adapt to our changing lives and times. It causes us to seek new experiences, and to feel comfortable in any new situation. It calms the adrenal glands and eliminates panic or uneasiness. Its vibration may fill in for our missing beats, and its elements, iron and calcium, can radiate for us a feeling of well-being that makes it unnecessary to impress others with our own opinions. This gem is sometimes prescribed to help eliminate stubbornness and an overly opinionated projection. It can soften the heart chakra.

In the yellow tinge, the vibration is of a very positive, optimistic outlook. It is often prescribed for the negative self-image.

The brownish vibration is for a settling-in calmness. The psychic and color properties are very minute but absolutely essential to the total formula.

The lack of hardness says, psychically, that the green garnet offers a softer vibration, with less strictness than the Emerald. The use of this gem would be suggested when the more modified vibrations from Saturn would be needed to reestablish order that has been lost. (Sometimes, through trauma, an otherwise disciplined personality will suffer disorientation.) The Green Garnet meditation is designed for relief of pressure in such situations.

GREEN GARNET MEDITATION

If the Green Garnet can be used for seven minutes in meditation every day and worn as jewelry with the full understanding of its properties, it will improve problems affecting the back and spine, deposits in the joints, and spastic colon, all of which are directly caused by incorrect mind-set.

The Green Garnet is vibrating at a rate of change that helps us to adapt to our changing lives and times. It causes us to seek new experiences and to feel comfortable in any new situation.

This gem is sometimes prescribed to help eliminate stubbornness and an overly opionionated personality. Regular meditation will:

1. Make us flexible to change
2. Eliminate pessimism
3. Relieve tension
4. Affect body chemical distribution

Method

Lie down on the floor on your back. Hold the Green Garnet in your palm and gaze at it for one full minute.

Place the Green Garnet against the . . .

SOLAR PLEXUS (near waist): Cover with palm, repeat seven times . . . "This Green Garnet is vibrating to help me adapt to changes with comfort."

HEART: Cover with palm, repeat seven times . . . "This Green Garnet is vibrating to eliminate pessimistic thoughts and words."

FOREHEAD: ("third eye"): Cover with palm, repeat seven times . . . "This Green Garnet is vibrating to relax my nerve centers."

The Blue-Indigo Ray Uranus

LAPIS LAZULI ◆ SAPPHIRE ◆ TURQUOISE

"Intuition is our contact between conscious and subconscious. We do whatever things come spontaneously to us, then suddenly we are aware of thought. Intuition is really the key to thinking."

—Buckminster Fuller

▲▲▲

The blue ray of Uranus enters our body through the pituitary, which is the "mind power center of imagination." There are several blue gemstones that are activated by Uranus, each having a different spiritual, mental, and physical effect on humans due to their chemical elements. This difference causes the molecular structure of the crystal to vibrate at different rates, providing individual messages, protections, stimulants, tranquilizers, and suggestions.

The planet Uranus was first observed in our solar system

on March 13, 1781. Astrologers paired it with Aquarius, described by ancient Eastern mystics as the root of intelligence representing the higher self. It is the part of the mind capable of sensing the causal nature whose impulse is toward investigation, absorption, and sensation. The abstract meaning is the power to express ideals.

Egyptian astrologers gave Uranus to the sign of Aquarius because of their affinity with each other. Two parallel, wavy lines were the glyph designated to signify Aquarius. Misinterpreted as water, these parallel lines of force actually represent vibration or electricity; Uranus is known as the electric planet. As an air sign related to the higher mind, Aquarius resonates with the invisible vibrations of the Universal Consciousness transmitted through Uranus.

Uranus affects our higher Mental Body. It knows no boundaries, manifesting itself in all areas of life, including the humanities, science, and art. Uranus, working through the right brain, gives us the ability to know things intuitively without needing Mercury's reason and logic.

Since we know that the orbit of Uranus around the Sun is eighty-four years, we know that when it enters Earth's cycle, it does so in a different sign of the Zodiac each time. During each transit of a sign by Uranus, a different aspect of electricity is discovered or applied.

Between 1814 and 1820, when Uranus was in the sign of Sagittarius, as it has been again during the last nine years (1981–1988), many inventions and theories pertaining to light and electricity were discovered. Berzelius theorized the chemical actions of electricity, H. Davy invented the miner's safety lamp, and Ampère discovered the laws of electrodynamic action.

In 1832, as Uranus transited through Aquarius, Samuel Morse invented the telegraph. In a more recent transit through Aquarius, Niels Bohr discovered atomic structure (1913), and Einstein broke new ground with his theory of relativity (1916).

When Uranus passed through Aries between 1844 and 1851, Thomas Edison and Alexander Graham Bell were born (1847). William Roentgen, discoverer of the X ray, was born in 1845 and George Westinghouse in 1846. The Russian scientist Pavlov, born in 1849, discovered the psychological "conditioned reflex" that led to widespread experimental research on the electrical pathways within the brain.

The second transit of Uranus through Aries between 1927 and 1935 saw the discovery of alpha waves and the beginning of "brain scan" equipment. The analog computer was invented in 1930, and the cyclotron, one of the basic tools of nuclear science, was invented in 1931.

According to Elman Bakcher's *Studies in Astrology*, from the Rosicrucian Fellowship, Uranus always acts to shatter and decrystallize the no longer needed, so that the fullness of progress on all planets may be revealed and realized. The significance of Uranus' appearance in our galaxy in 1781 can be ascertained by the American Revolution's occurring at that time, after which a new world was created.

Uranus is now in the sign of "higher mind," Sagittarius, the sign associated with publishing, education, law, religion, and long journeys. In this position Uranus practically guarantees revolution in all these areas.

Religion and law are certainly due for a breakup of old patterns with avant-garde theories emerging to replace them. The computer has revolutionized publishing with the word processing machine and has enhanced education with its use in classrooms all over America.

Uranus continues to exert its influence on Earth, penetrating deep into the mineral-crystal center, blasting away all the unnecessary psychic baggage that we carry. Its shocking vibrations transmitted to human beings through Uranus blue rays will stimulate deeper thinking so that shallow understandings can be replaced with wisdom applicable to daily life.

LAPIS LAZULI

CHEMICAL COMPOSITION: $(Na,Ca)_4(SO_4,S,Cl)$ $(AlSiO_4)_3$ (tektosilicate group)
CRYSTAL SYSTEM: Isometric crystal formation very rare. Well-formed dodecahedrons.
RAY: Blue Indigo
PLANET: Uranus
POWER CENTER OF IMAGINATION
HEALTH FACTORS: Right brain, calms the adrenal glands
PSYCHIC QUALITIES: Courage, safety, protection, raises the Kundalini

General Science

The name *Lapis Lazuli* is from the ancient Persian *lazhu-ward*. In its best form it is an intense rich blue, very often containing pyrite (gold flecks), or calcite (a white vein). On a scale of 1 to 10, it measures 5½ in hardness. It is sometimes called lazurite, which is the main ingrediant.

Lazurite is found in Afghanistan, the USSR, Chile, and in Colorado and California in the United States. The most beautiful is from Afghanistan.

History, Myth, and Magic

One of the oldest known gemstones, Lapis Lazuli was used extensively by the Egyptians for thousands of years, before the Old Testament of the Hebrew Bible was written. It is mentioned in the book of Exodus (28:15–30) as one of twelve precious stones to be built into the religious vestments of the Hebrew high priests. At that time, the Hebrew word was *sappir* and has often been confused by translations as Sapphire, since both gems are blue. However, the crystal systems are entirely different, as well as vital elements. The vibrations are consequently very individual.

The Babylonians, writing before the Hebrews and the Egyptians, believed the Lapis to be a cure for melancholy and fever. There are several pieces of limestone in the collection of the Metropolitan Museum of Art in New York that are inscribed with Egyptian writings from approximately 1600 B.C. These writings have been translated and describe the treatment of hysteria with Lapis Lazuli.

The Egyptians used the Lapis extensively for amulets and fetishes. Its relative softness made it easy to carve into the shapes of animals, insects, flowers, and hearts. Graves have been found containing Lapis carvings dating around 2000 B.C. In the Egyptian *Book of the Dead*, it was ordered that the 166th chapter written in 4400 B.C. be engraved on a Lapis heart.

The rituals for burial and afterlife were very important to the Egyptians. The 26th chapter of the *Book of the Dead* was to be engraved on a scarab and placed on the body in a separate container to protect the heart during its astral journey. An eye carved of Lapis and engraved with the 140th chapter, concerning Truth, was worn by the highest priest of Egypt.

Trading brought the Lapis to China, where it had religious significance when worn by the emperor for services in the Temple of Heaven. In all the intellectually advanced societies of that time, the Lapis was understood to have a powerful vibration and was used by leaders.

Leonardo da Vinci used Lapis crushed for his ultramarine-blue oil paints, as did most artists of his time. This has a special significance in the effect that his paintings have upon the viewer. It also explains the protection that his paintings have received throughout five hundred years of war and destruction. It is only in this century that synthetic coloring has been manufactured.

Even in these modern times the mining of Lapis is very

primitive in Afghanistan, where the highest quality and most beautiful specimens are found. The natives build fires under the limestone cliffs where the veins of Lapis develop. When the rocks are hot, cold water is thrown onto them, causing large chunks to crack off. This slow method has kept the value of the stone at a higher level. The price of Lapis is rising today because the Russian invasion of Afghanistan has practically stopped mining.

There are some fine deposits in Russia, and Catherine II was one of the royal family to use large slabs of Lapis in decorating walls and pillars of her palaces.

Unfortunately, imitation Lapis is now marketed, such as blue-dyed chalcedony. A synthetic Lapis has been manufactured in France that even contains the pyrite flakes most often used as identification of the original gem. Even glass is used to imitate Lapis. It would be wise not to purchase Lapis from any other than a reputable gemologist.

Healing Secrets

The deep, rich blue of the Lapis is of a very quieting origin. In owning and working with a Lapis, the adrenal glands are tranquilized. This causes acids that are harmful to the stomach and intestines to flow only when necessary for digestion. Therefore, if a Lapis is chosen or suggested, it will be effective as a deterrent to ulcers and forms of intestinal cancer. It will calm a nervous stomach and aid digestion.

If you are a healer and wish to use Lapis as an aid, hold it enclosed within your own hand while working with the other hand. It will keep the healer steady and strong.

Psychic Strengths

The qualities of the geometric formula of the Lapis Lazuli/ Lazurite cause a vibration of the mind to see and comprehend things that would otherwise have been passed over or ignored. It vibrates alertness. It brings to the holder the message, "Pay attention to what is happening around you . . . open your eyes and see."

The second main axis in this crystal has a vibrational formula to raise the sexual urge from purely animal to the level of love. This energy is the strongest force known to man. If it is correctly directed, it results in great genius. If it is misdirected, it is a destroyer. In modern language, the Lapis Lazuli says "get your mind above your belt."

The Lapis, because of its effects on the alert mind, offers a more relaxed and secure inner emotion. The aggravation of mistakes and accidents will be minimized as the holder daily becomes more alert. The aggravation of preoccupation with sexual encounter will allow more inspired mind work and job advancement. The color is one that eliminates nervousness and anxiety.

It is also most useful in warding off psychic attack. The Babylonians and Egyptians, advanced in technology beyond our level, knew this. The wearing of a Lapis over the heart can protect against all evil thought forms that may be picked up from others, or deliberately sent to us by another.

The vibration that prevents psychic attack is a second note in the Lapis geometry. As previously mentioned, the second vibration raises the ability to love from the erotic level to the sensitive heart level. In the case of anyone who is "waiting" for love, this vibration will raise their awareness to the love that already exists. With a stimulated heart they will be able to recognize and respond to that higher aspect of love. This does not discount the sexual, but elevates the spirit of each.

The study of the psychic properties and use of gems, including Lapis, was most probably carried around the Earth by the survivors from Atlantis. It was known and used by Sumerians, Babylonians, Egyptians, Hebrews, Indians, Chinese, and all the ancient wisdom cultures. The fact that only nine hundred years ago the Church in Europe put a stop to the use of gems does not discount the truth as it has been recounted in both the Old and New Testaments of the Bible.

Since Lapis Lazuli has one of the *earliest* recorded histories, archaeologists easily recognize the significant role that it had psychically and spiritually in these ancient, advanced civilizations.

LAPIS LAZULI MEDITATION

As the receiver of Uranus's blue rays of wisdom and balance, Lapis helps channel the Kundalini energy. Originating at the base of the spine and rising upward to the skull, this electric energy (pictured in Eastern philosophy as a serpent) stimulates the creative mind.

If the Kundalini is not consciously focused, it becomes base animal sexual urge. This invisible energy within every human is no more mysterious than radio or television. It is always there and always active whether we use it or not. Meditating with Lapis will show immediate creative results and will:

1. Vibrate alertness to the senses
2. Protect against negative thought forms
3. Raise the creative urge from physical to mental
4. Calm the adrenals, aid digestion, and protect the stomach

Method

Lie down on the floor on your back. Hold the Lapis in your palm and gaze at it for one full minute.

Place the Lapis against the . . .
SOLAR PLEXUS (near waist): Cover with palm, repeat seven times . . . "This Lapis is calming, aiding, and protecting my emotions."
HEART: Cover with palm, repeat seven times . . . "This Lapis repels any negative thought forms."
FOREHEAD ("third eye"): Cover with palm, repeat seven times . . . "This Lapis is alerting my senses to my own good."

BLUE SAPPHIRE

CHEMICAL COMPOSITION: Al_2O_3 (aluminum oxide)
CRYSTAL SYSTEM: Hexagonal—scalenohedral
BLUE/INDIGO RAY
PLANET: Uranus
POWER CENTER OF IMAGINATION
HEALTH FACTOR: Blood circulation, pituitary balancing
PSYCHIC QUALITIES: Alertness, overcoming sadness

General Science

The true color of the Sapphire is blue, though it may also be a multitude of other colors as well: red, yellow, violet, green, and a beautiful hair-brown color that Venetian painters liked to use with golden light shining through it. Sapphires change color by artificial light at times, and those of the clearest blue come from Ceylon. These are of pure alumina.

When the Sapphire is examined with a spectograph or an X ray, the interior crystal formation is always a hexagonal dipyramid—perfectly geometrical, never deviating. It is second in hardness only to the diamond. The finest blue gem Sapphires occur in Kashmir, North India, and even though there are very few found there now, the finest Sapphires are referred to as "Kashmiris." Other gem quality Sapphires are found in Madagascar, South Africa, Mozambique, Burma, and Ceylon. In the United States the largest deposits are found in Georgia and North Carolina. They are also found in Montana as water-worn pebbles by the Missouri River. In California, small well-formed crystals can be found in Riverside, San Bernardino, and San Diego.

History, Myth, and Magic

The Sapphire is one of the oldest known stones in written history. Both Sapphire and Ruby come from the same family, known as corundum.

The Sapphire and the Ruby are identically the same stone. Both have the same hardness, composition, and electrical properties, but they differ in the amount of color mineral within each. Though the Lapis Lazuli is remarkably similar in color to the Sapphire, its composition is different from that of the Sapphire, and the Ruby for that matter.

In the South Kensington Museum in London, there is a Sapphire of a peculiar tint. In daylight this stone is a blue color. But in artificial light, it has a violet hue and resembles an Amethyst.

In the eighteenth century Mme. de Genlis wrote a story called *Le Saphire Merveilleux* in which the Sapphire was used as a test of female virtue. Any change of color indicated unfaithfulness by its wearer. The woman whose virtue was in question was made to wear the stone for three daylight hours as a test of her faithfulness. Often when the test was administered, however, the subject would not fare well if the test begun in daylight ended in candlelight. The artificial light would change the stone to purple, much to the chagrin of the hopeless subject of inquiry.

The story of the Russian Grand Duke Sergius is interesting. When he was assassinated (March 6, 1905) in a bomb explosion, an unusual stone completely black in color was discovered among his personal effects. It proved to be the Duke's Sapphire ring, which had lost its color as a result of the method of execution, the bomb's intense light.

The Morgan-Tiffany Collection in the American Museum of Natural History is the home of the wonderful "asteria" (Star Sapphire), which is called the Star of India. The history of this magnificent gem spans three centuries. After its many wanderings, it has found a final resting place in this great museum. It weighs 543 carats.

During the Middle Ages extraordinary virtues were attributed to the Sapphire, which was believed to have sexual distinctions. The masculine gender correlated to the pale-blue Sapphire, while the feminine gender corresponded to the dark-blue variety. From a medical perspective, they "fortified the heart, counteracted the effects of poisons, purified the blood, and dried up ulcers on the eyes."

Healing Secrets

The blue ray enters the body by the pituitary gland in the head. Of the twelve basic chakras or mind power centers of the body, the pituitary is the "power center of imagination."

Dr. Phineas P. Quimby, one of the world's foremost enlightened spiritual physicians, told Americans of the nineteenth century: "Imagination is probably the most powerful faculty of the human mind. Thousands of practical men today know that what the mind images becomes experience and fact."

To heal the body, the imagination in the mind must first form a mental picture of health. Once you have seen the result you wish to attain, you have already willed a means that will take you to the result. We built our own bodies by choosing the genetic linkup of chromosomes and molecules present in the mixture that was made by our mother and father. We have the ability to further influence the building and repair of this same body. To aid in this creative process, the light inside the human mind that is the Divine creative imagination lives in the pituitary gland in the brain. If there is any disruption of the pituitary function brought about by consistently unhealthy thought or emotions of anger, resentment, depression, jealousy, fear, etc., there can be no light.

One of the most common physical ailments that reflects unhealthy thinking is arthritis. In a very large percentage of those suffering with this crippling disease, psychologists have found patients holding a deep-seated anger or resentment against someone or something from the past.

Psychic Strengths

In her book *Spiritual Value of Gem Stones*, Lenora Huett states that the clear blue Sapphire works more efficiently with the invisible mental body, and the Star Sapphire works with the chakra centers of the etheric body.

Julia Lorusso and Joel Glick collaborated on a "channeled" book in 1976 entitled *The Therapeutic Use of Gems and Minerals.* In this writing, they specifically mention Sapphire of the darkest blue, working on the indigo ray from Saturn, to eliminate confusion and illusion.

Confusion and illusion are the key words to diagnosis of many illnesses. It is widely accepted by metaphysicians that the common cold is often a result of confusion and that the manic-depressive suffers from illusion.

Whether the Sapphire is working on the blue or indigo ray, the vibration raises the consciousness through imagination, that is, to visualize, "see" the physical body healthful and whole.

Properties of a Star Sapphire

Like the Ruby, the Star Sapphire is not a clear or transparent gem. Trapped inside is titanium dioxide (rutile), which causes the light refraction to form a six-pointed star when the Sapphire is polished "en cabochon."

The appearance of this star psychically represents the New Age, rebirth and a new perception, as the Star of Bethlehem heralded a new age of thought.

To properly meditate upon the Star Sapphire, gaze upon the star for one full minute. Then, follow each ray from the source to the end for one full minute each.

When this seven-minute meditation is completed, write down any thoughts that come into your mind. They will seem like new thoughts to you because your new perception will cause you to accept them in a new way. As your inner eyesight is stimulated, you will see before you what you need to know.

CAUTION: Star Sapphires are being produced chemically in man-made stones. They are very beautiful and not inexpensive. However, their vibrations will not be the same as a natural cosmic Sapphire.

BLUE SAPPHIRE MEDITATION

To heal the body, the imagination must first form a mental picture of health. Sapphire, working through the blue and indigo rays, vibrates to raise the consciousness through imagination by visualization, actually "seeing" the physical body as well and whole.

Uranus, ruler of the sign Aquarius, governs the ankles and circulation of blood. Working with the Sapphire benefits these areas of the body.

Working in the emotional realm, the Sapphire is effective in healing depression. Many personalities benefit from the "zap" that is felt by anyone using this gem, as it actually jolts the mind-set of sadness or melancholy right into conscious awareness. This shocking vibration will stimulate deeper thinking so that shallow understandings can be replaced with wisdom applicable to daily life.

The Sapphire-Uranus gem-ray connection is sometimes so powerful that it acts like a cosmic "slap in the face" to a hysterical person. Holding and contemplating a Sapphire every day will accomplish the following:

1. Replace sadness or melancholy with a feeling of light and joy
2. Change shallow thinking into deeper, more meaningful understanding
3. Quiet overemotional irritation or nervousness
4. Elevate boring fundamentalism to a higher plane of imagination

Method

Lie down on the floor on your back. Hold the Sapphire in your palm and gaze at it for one full minute.

Place the Sapphire against the . . .

186 / THE HEALING COLOR CONNECTION

SOLAR PLEXUS (near waist): Cover with palm, repeat seven times . . . "This Sapphire is vibrating to 'zap' sadness!"

HEART: Cover with palm, repeat seven times . . . "This Sapphire is vibrating to increase the positive mental picture I have of myself."

FOREHEAD ("third eye"): Cover with palm, repeat seven times . . . "This Sapphire is vibrating to break up old patterns of negativity."

TURQUOISE

CHEMICAL COMPOSITION: $CuAl_6(OH)_2/PO_4)_4 \cdot 4H_2O$ (copper containing basic aluminum phosphate)
CRYSTAL SYSTEM: Triclinic
BLUE RAY
PLANET: Uranus
POWER CENTER OF IMAGINATION
HEALTH FACTOR: Visualizing desired state of perfect health
PSYCHIC QUALITIES: Ancient wisdom, creativity, courage to speak the truth, imagination

General Science

This stone, the oldest known to recorded history, is colored opaque sky-blue to blue-green. The truth of its real atomic composition was not discovered until 1911. Up until actual crystals were found in the United States, it was believed to be amorphous.

The stone is most often found containing a matrix, foreign veins of brown (limonite), dark gray (sandstone), or black (Jasper). It is very unusual to find pure pale robin's-egg-blue Turquoise. The very cleanest and best stones in the world are mined in northeast Iran. Its habit of growth is in very dense form, filling fissures in other rocks with its grape or nodule formation.

The color is adversely affected by perspiration, hand oils, and exposure to light or heat. The color change will be to greens. It is often found growing with Malachite or Chrysocolla, which are basically more green.

It is an easy gem to carve and shape, as the hardness on the Mohs' scale of 1 to 10 is 5 or 6.

Turquoise is mined today in Afghanistan, Australia, Tibet, Israel, Tanzania, Chile, Brazil, and the southwestern United States, with rare crystals from Virginia.

History, Myth, and Magic

The spelling of "turquoise" is from the French, as they called it *pierre turquoise* or stone of Turkey. Its origin, however, is not in that country. Istanbul, then the capital of Turkey, was the trading center of gems traveling from Iran, Afghanistan, Tibet, and various other Mideastern and Eastern countries to Europe. The Turquoise most in demand came from Persia, as it was the most pure sky blue with the fewest veins of matrix or other impurities. It reached its peak of trading during the Ottoman Empire.

Long before then, however, this stone was being mined in the Sinai Peninsula by the Egyptians.

The astounding similarity between the carved Turquoise found in ancient Egyptian tombs and the graves of North American Indians has led many archaeologists to speculate on the possibility of a common background for the races. The believers in a lost continent sunk beneath the Atlantic Ocean often link the migration of the original human species across America before it reached Africa, India, and the Middle East.

In the thirteenth century the stone took on the French name of Turquoise. At that time Turquoise was said to protect against injury from falling, whether riding or walking, as long as the gem was carried on the person.

In the fourteenth century, the *lapidaire* of Sir John Mandeville assigned protection to horses to keep them from falling, or from exhaustion. It is supposed that he got this information from the Turks, who often put Turquoise amulets on the bridles of their horses.

Anselmus de Boot was a court physician in 1609 to Rudolf II of Germany. Very involved with using the gems in healing, he wrote a treatise called *Gemmarum et Lapidum Historia*. He mentioned Turquoise in several instances as he was particularly involved with a piece that had been given to him by his father. It was a very pale stone (probably having lost its moisture), and after De Boot had had it carved with his family crest and began to wear it in a ring, it regained its color. The same ring was broken on two occasions when De Boot accidentally fell. In both instances, his body could have been seriously injured but was not. Being a religious man, he was convinced that the spirit of angels penetrates certain gems.

Mme. Catulle Mendes, a French literary figure of the 1700s, was convinced that her jewels each had a personality. She explained that if she left her Turquoises alone in a drawer too long, they became as pale as death. She would wear all of her rings together as much as possible so none of them would feel slighted.

Healing Secrets

Because the Turquoise is conducting ray-waves from the planet Uranus through the pituitary gland in the head, it directly affects our "power center of imagination." To make a mental image takes the ability to "see" what is not physically there to see. In medical or physiological terms, there are twenty times as many nerves running from the eyes to the brain as there are from the ears to the brain. Seeing is more important than hearing. You can hear my words, but if I show you a picture, you are more likely to remember what I say.

By picturing yourself in perfect health, you can actually rearrange the molecular structure of certain less well areas in your body. This allows your naturally perfect body to reform its own cells, so that organic healing occurs.

The creative act of visualization is an (electric) current or wave that emanates from the brain at such a rate that it causes matter to be moved. If there is a concentration on a desired state of health, if a mental picture is held consistently, the Universal Law of Attraction makes the molecules move into a healthful state.

This power of imagination is triggered by the use of the Turquoise, as it transmits ray-waves from Uranus, the planet of unique, imaginative, higher mind right-brain activity. The stone itself has no magic power. It is an aid for concentration of Cosmic power. The person who desires healing must dedicate a period of time each day to work with the transmitter to concentrate on a visual image of the healthy working part of the body in question.

To aid in this process, it is necessary to know exactly how the portion of the body in question appears in a healthful condition. The anatomical section of an encyclopedia will have illustrations of this specific area. Study the picture until a clear visualization can be manifested with the eyes closed. Imagine yourself looking inside your own body until you find the area in question, and immediately picture this area in perfect working order.

This takes dedication of specific time daily without interruption. The amount of improvement depends upon the amount of time given to the image. The Turquoise can only be used on the self in this manner. Another person cannot do our imaging for us, nor can we do it for another.

Psychic Strengths

Turquoise is a carrier of ancient wisdom and knowledge. Unconcerned with time and space, it carries knowledge and wisdom of all the ages. The Turquoise, because it is a conductor of the electric planet, can reveal to us all of the future as well as the past. Turquoise receives the ray-waves of Uranus in a universal, impersonal way. In other words, it is not a respecter of persons. The Turquoise simply states the facts. It is a record of past, present, and future. There is no judgment in Turquoise. Neither education nor IQ impresses the Turquoise; it will divulge the facts to anyone who wishes to know them. Each person who uses the Turquoise in this manner will receive information according to their ability to assimilate.

Uranus, operating in the blue ray, is electric. "Electric blue" is the color seen when an arc of electricity is produced. The blue ray, according to esoteric historians such as Alice Baily, is the sixth ray of love wisdom. All blue gems and minerals are transmitting the blue ray in their various capacities. Turquoise is the impersonal love wisdom, in that it gives to all without judgment.

Impersonal love is altruism. It gives without any expectation of reward or return. That is the epitome of wisdom. We have problems with this impersonal love because we are so rooted to the physical that our left-brain, logical mind is telling us that we must receive something in return if we are to give love away.

However, we constantly receive love through physical blessings. The rain falls on the just and the unjust. The rainbow is enjoyed by the believer and the nonbeliever alike. Every aspect of beauty and peace is available to both the faithful and the infidel. Nothing is withheld from us for we are loved without question of our worth or deservedness.

TURQUOISE MEDITATION

Because the Turquoise is conducting ray-waves from the planet Uranus through the pituitary gland in the head, it directly affects our "power center of imagination."

Visualizing a picture of yourself in perfect health can actually rearrange the molecular structure of unwell areas of the body. This allows the naturally perfect body to be released so that organic healing occurs.

The Turquoise itself has no magic power but acts to aid Cosmic Currents. The person who desires healing must dedicate a period of time each day to working with this transmitter by concentrating on a visual image of the healthy, working body.

For those who truly want to teach, Turquoise is a carrier of ancient wisdom and knowledge. There is no judgment in Turquoise. It acts to:

1. Carry ancient wisdom and the truth of ages
2. Give confidence to speak knowledge
3. Affect the mind power of imagination
4. Perfect pituitary function

Method

Lie down on the floor on your back. Hold the Turquoise in your palm and gaze at it for one full minute.

Place the Turquoise against the . . .

SOLAR PLEXUS (near waist): Cover with palm, repeat seven times . . . "This Turquoise is vibrating to give me the ancient wisdoms."

HEART: Cover with palm, repeat seven times . . . "This Turquoise gives me confidence to speak knowledge."

FOREHEAD ("third eye"): Cover with palm, repeat seven times . . . "This Turquoise is vibrating to open my power center of imagination."

Venus
Light Blue Ray

AQUAMARINE ◆ BLUE TOPAZ

"Love gives naught but itself, and takes not
but from itself. Love possesses not nor would
it be possessed . . . and think not you can direct the course of love, for love, if it finds you
worthy, directs your course."

—**Kahlil Gibran**

▲▲▲

The "power center of will" is located in the part of the
forebrain surrounding the pineal gland. It is through this
point that the light blue ray-wave from Venus enters and
aids our creative process.

The vibrations or transmissions from Venus are basically
described as harmony, unison, and relatedness. These rays
increase our ability to attract others to us in friendship,
partnership, and close relationships. Venus vibrations affect our social instincts and activities. Our awareness in the
areas of art and beauty is also heightened.

Venus is one of our nearest neighbors. We have been receiving its subliminal assistance from the earliest times. For instance, the appreciation of art and beauty has introduced culture into our civilized world. And the evolution into monogamous marriage was inspired by the ray-waves emitted from Venus through its inherent energy of partnership and cooperation. The very survival and advancement of civilization have been dependent on these messages.

Astronomers and astrologers alike have regarded Venus as a sister to Earth because of their similarity in size, volume, mass, density, and gravity. However, Venus rotates in the opposite direction from Earth, with one day equivalent to almost a year on Earth. Surrounded as it is by a heavy cloud layer, all of our information about Venus has been received from radar, radio waves, and unmanned space satellite probes.

The glyph astrologers use to designate Venus comes directly from an ancient Egyptian insignia called the ankh, a symbol popularized by the "flower children" during the peace and love movement of the late sixties and early seventies.

To the Hindu, Venus was born of a lotus from the sea. The Greeks also depicted Venus emerging from water, symbolizing the ocean of space.

The creative artists of the world respond to the Venusian vibration. In an astrological chart the planet Venus placement describes the feminine attributes, which include loving and creative qualities.

AQUAMARINE

(Beryl Group)
CHEMICAL COMPOSITION: $Al_2Be_3(Si_6O_{18})$ (aluminum beryllium silicate)
CRYSTAL SYSTEM: Hexagonal (trigonal)
LIGHT BLUE RAY (Also includes pink in the spectrum of light we have not learned to see)
PLANET: Venus
POWER CENTER OF WILL
HEALTH FACTOR: Pineal gland, right brain, kidneys
PSYCHIC QUALITIES: Anxiety relief, peace of mind

General Science

The Aquamarine is a sister to the Emerald, both being from the beryl family. The color of Aquamarine is the source of its name, derived from Latin meaning "water of the sea." The gem is a clear, transparent blue-green color—the darker the color, the more valuable the stone. The color-producing pigment is iron. There is speculation that a rare metal, scandium, may also affect the color. Lighter stones are heated to change their color.

The double refraction of light from different angles within the crystal causes it to reflect two different colors, blue and green. On occasion, fine, hollow rods become included during the formation of crystals. When this occurs, the stone can be cut "en cabochon" rather than faceted. This cut displays a cat's-eye effect or asterism with a six-rayed star. Some of these appear almost black when viewed from the top but clear when viewed from the side.

On a hardness scale of 1 to 10, Aquamarine measures 7½–8. However, it is brittle and may fracture in spite of its relative hardness.

Aquamarine deposits are found on almost every continent, but the most important are located in Brazil. The

well-known Russian deposits in the Ural Mountains appear
to be worked out. Other deposits of smaller importance
are located in Australia, Burma, Sri Lanka, India, Kenya,
and South Africa. In the United States, discoveries have
been made in California, Colorado, Connecticut, Maine,
and North Carolina.

This gem is often found in very large crystals. In 1910,
a two hundred forty-three pound Aquamarine was found
in Brazil, the largest gem-quality crystal ever found. It was
eighteen inches long and fifteen inches in diameter. Classified as semiprecious, a fine clear Aquamarine, however,
may be more valuable than a flawed Emerald.

History, Myth, and Magic

The Egyptian amulets of the XII Dynasty (circa 2000 B.C.)
that have been recovered include Aquamarine cut into the
forms of animals. An ancient statue in Alicante, Spain,
dating back to 2500 B.C., is supposedly the Egyptian goddess Isis. Carved upon the pedestal is a list of jewels given
as a religious sacrifice to the goddess by an Egyptian grand-
mother, Fabis Fabiana, to save her granddaughter. They
included two ankle bracelets of Aquamarines.

Greek goldsmiths of the period before the conquest of
Rome used Aquamarines in their jewelry. The gemstones
were brought to them from the Far East, Russia, and Persia
by camel caravan across Arabia, and then by ship to their
ports on the Mediterranean. Some large light-colored stones,
up to one hundred carats in size, are displayed in the most
dramatic jewelry ever made.

Around A.D. 400 a treatise in the Greek lapidary described the jewels used by sailors to protect themselves at
sea. Ships were rather primitive and the Mediterranean
was a particularly stormy sea, so it is not difficult to imagine

that marine safety was pretty chancy at best. Aquamarine was chosen to banish fear.

A dream book, attributed to or called *Achametis*, written in the eighth century and probably Arabic in origin, states that if an Aquamarine appears in a dream, it symbolizes new friends. In A.D. 1220, Arnoldus Saxo combined the works of Aristotle, Marbodus, Exax, and Isidorus to compile yet another essay on gems. He added the Aquamarine and gave it the power to influence amiability in the personality.

Healing Secrets

The Aquamarine vibration has a special effect on the pineal body or gland. This is a small, reddish cone-shaped body on the dorsal portion of the brain of all vertebrates. Its function is obscure, however, research has discovered that in some species it is connected to a median eye-like structure on the dorsal surface of the head. In metaphysical terms, it is called the "third eye" and is located in the center of the forehead. When an Aquamarine is suggested for meditation, it is an indication that the pineal gland is not functioning to capacity and needs to have its vibration raised. It is in this area that the judgment and perception of situations or persons is psychically perceived. When the pineal is not operating correctly, there is a tendency toward naïveté, immature gullibility, and openness to constant disappointment.

In the mathematical predictability of the workings of the brain, the pituitary gland is triggered when the pineal is working properly. This pituitary adjusts itself and correctly measures the liquid enzymes and hormones to be distributed in the body. An overall improvement in physical well-being occurs. It is not a dramatic change, but gentle and noticeable. The person for whom Aquamarine is recommended may already have a fairly well-balanced psychosomatic nature and only needs this light vibration to become totally balanced.

Psychic Strengths

The Aquamarine is often recommended for meditation by persons of a quiet nature and soft voice because it has a very gentle vibration. Often these outward signs are misleading to others who may not detect the inner strength and determination. There is often a very aesthetic mindset, somewhat idealistic and very creative, in the person for whom Aquamarine is suggested.

Because of the quiet method of being that one has chosen to display to the world, there is often an inward conflict of mind. The person may be easily startled by changing events and may become inwardly nervous and distraught. This sensitive nature can be compared to that of a fawn, sleeping in the woods, who jumps and darts about frantically with the snap of a twig. The Aquamarine vibration can return the calm, inward strength that is actually present and part of the original makeup of the person.

In personal relationships this kind and peaceful personality may become dismayed at violent or inconsiderate actions of others. This causes an inner storm, because there is within this quiet personality a violence of its own, an inner and hidden rebellion or revolt against an aggressor. If this is allowed to go unchecked, the pituitary gland malfunctions, causing overdoses of enzymes and hormones to be dumped into the system in poisonous doses. Since it is not possible for this personality to display such violent emotion outwardly, it is necessary to have the emotion released. Meditation with the Aquamarine can release and adjust these vibrations.

The creative processes can also be heightened and released in a more mature manner. As meditation improves discernment, the imagination grows away from impractical childish creativity into gainful production.

AQUAMARINE MEDITATION

The Aquamarine is often recommended for meditation by persons of a quiet nature and soft voice because of the gem's gentle vibration. Often these outward signs are misleading to others who do not detect the inner strength and determination.

There is often a very aesthetic mind-set that is somewhat idealistic and very creative in the person for whom Aquamarine is suggested.

Since the vibrational message of Aquamarine is "peace," the person using the gem may also send peace to another. After meditating to insure one's own peace of mind, concentrate on the other person for a few moments. While contemplating a picture of a peaceful lake at sunrise placed over the person's image, speak the words, "My peace I send you." Neither time nor distance have any constraint on this treatment.

In all historical references to the Aquamarine, it has been linked with water. For this reason it is recommended that water become a form of therapy to increase the well-being of anyone choosing an Aquamarine.

1. Have a fountain or pool of water in or near the living quarters.
2. Use cassette recordings of streams, rain, or ocean waves for relaxation.
3. Place paintings or pictures of waves, waterfalls, or lakes where they can be viewed regularly.

4. Immerse the whole body in warm water when stress is detected.
5. Whenever possible, be near natural bodies of water.

Method

Lie down on the floor on your back. Hold the Aquamarine in your palm and gaze at it for one full minute.

Place the Aquamarine against the . . .

SOLAR PLEXUS (near waist): Cover with palm, repeat seven times . . . "This Aquamarine is vibrating to bring peace to my emotions."

HEART: Cover with palm, repeat seven times . . . "This Aquamarine is vibrating to bring peace to my heart."

FOREHEAD ("third eye"): Cover with palm, repeat seven times . . . "This Aquamarine is vibrating to bring me peace of mind."

BLUE TOPAZ

CHEMICAL COMPOSITION: $Al_2(SiO_4)(F,OH)_2$
BLUE RAY
PLANET: Venus (also Jupiter)
POWER CENTERS OF WILL AND ZEAL
HEALTH FACTORS: Thyroid balancing down
PSYCHIC QUALITIES: Calmness, hypertension relief
BENEFITS OF MEDITATION: Choosing a Blue Topaz
   indicates the wearer or holder is in need of relaxation
   and that an overstimulated nervous system must be
   calmed. More about this gem is written in the chapter
   dealing with its ruling planet, Uranus.

The element present in the crystal structure of the Topaz
that changes its color from yellow to blue also opens its
vibrations to the ray-waves from Venus.
   Although the Blue Topaz is influenced by the feminine
vibration from Venus, it is ruled by the masculine rays and
description of Jupiter, giving it a double vibration of will
and zeal.
   Basically then, the Blue Topaz will increase interest in
the higher ideals of life. It promotes the spiritual understanding necessary to get moving in the direction of self-
improvement, with determination, awakened consciousness and peace of mind.
   This psychic combination is rare. Persons who are ready
for this gem have great potential toward soul evolution.
Meditation with Blue Topaz will achieve the following:
   1. Calm the nervous system
   2. Promote higher ideals
   3. Stimulate self-improvement
   4. Strengthen and awaken consciousness

Method

Lie down on the floor on your back, hold the Blue Topaz in your palm and gaze at it for one full minute.

Place the Blue Topaz against the . . .

SOLAR PLEXUS (near waist): Cover with palm, repeat seven times . . . "This Blue Topaz is vibrating to calm my nervous system."

HEART: Cover with palm, repeat seven times . . . "This Blue Topaz is vibrating to promote my positive self-improvement."

FOREHEAD ("third eye"): Cover with palm, repeat seven times . . . "This Blue Topaz is vibrating to help me remain focused with determination toward awakened consciousness in my daily life."

Mercury
The Violet Ray

AMETHYST

"As a people, we have become obsessed with health. There is something fundamentally, radically unhealthy about all this. . . . We have lost all confidence in the human body."

—Lewis Thomas
Past Dean at Yale Medical School
Chairman of the Department of Pathology and Medicine
President of Memorial Sloan-Kettering Cancer Center

▲▲▲

The violet gem-ray connection of Mercury that enters the body through the "power center of communication" located in the throat acts to aid all manner of mental activity, including physical communication of clear thought.

Closest to the Sun of all the planets, Mercury has always

been referred to as "the messenger of the gods." The hottest, quickest, and smallest of the Sun's cosmic family, Mercury rises and sets with the Sun and can only be viewed just after sunset or before sunrise. A month on Mercury is fifty-nine Earth days. Mercury has no moons and travels lightly and swiftly.

In astrology, the glyph for Mercury means "active intelligence." Thought to be a simplified version of the caduceus, a winged baton or rod entwined by two serpents, this glyph is the symbol associated with the medical profession today.

Mercury is the giver of the healing arts. As a messenger from the protector and proliferator of life, the Sun, Mercury bestows the physical knowledge, understanding, and wisdom necessary to promote and evolve physical life. The lower, earthly mind of logic and analysis is activated by Mercury.

As the transmitter of the spiritual to the material, Mercury brings to us the message of the teacher, communicator, writer, or healer from the Universal Consciousness. It helps us to know, understand, and communicate clearly. Mercury's function is to activate the left brain of humans. It separates the instinctual, animal, behavioral mind from reason, analysis, learning, and speech.

We possess the power of speech unknown to any other species. In the beginning was the Word. The spoken word is power, with vibrations that can change physical matter by changing brain waves.

Mercury helps us to know, understand, and communicate clearly the laws and practical side of the spiritual. It helps us to think clearly and logically about ourselves and those we wish to teach or heal. The cosmic ray-waves from Mercury also activate improvement and invention, causing the mind to seek and explore.

"There is something like telepathy going on around us, which I am convinced will ultimately be identified as ultra-ultra high frequency electromagnetic waves."

—**Buckminster Fuller**

▲▲▲

AMETHYST

CHEMICAL COMPOSITION: $SiO_2(Mn?)$ (tektosilicate ion)
CRYSTAL SYSTEM: Hexagonal (trigonal)
VIOLET RAY
PLANET: Mercury
POWER CENTER OF COMMUNICATION
HEALTH FACTOR: Protects throat, lungs, and respiratory system, healing others
PSYCHIC QUALITIES: Purifying and clarifying thoughts

General Science

Amethyst belongs to the family of Quartz. Although the word *quarz* is German, it is of uncertain origin. The element responsible for its pale to dark violet or purple color has not been absolutely determined. Manganese is a possibility, but really it remains more or less a mystery. The Amethyst is part of the hexagonal crystal system, most often found inside geodes. These are large stone "eggs" that formed when liquid filtered into the holes left by gas bubbles in hot lava, forming Amethyst crystals that grow pointing toward the center.

Amethyst, measuring 7 on the 1 to 10 Mohs' scale of hardness, is found in many places, including Nova Scotia and Ontario, Canada; Massachusetts, Connecticut, New Jersey, Pennsylvania, Virginia, North Carolina, South Carolina, Georgia, and Arizona; and Mexico. The largest geode ever found was in Minas Gerais, Brazil, measuring 33 feet long, 5½ feet wide, and 3 feet high. The best gem quality Amethyst is found in Uruguay. Korea has produced the largest single crystals, up to twelve inches in length. Rare twin crystals are found in Japan and are very collectible.

The best of a dark purplish-red Amethyst are called Siberian and are from the Ural Mountains in Russia, where they are no longer mined.

History, Myth, and Magic

The oldest written reference to the Amethyst is found in the Egyptian *Book of the Dead*. It was used as part of a necklace found on a mummy dated around 4000 B.C. The Egyptians used it in many amulet forms and executed many stone carvings depicting their history.

An ancient piece of Amethyst jewelry was found in an Egyptian burial tomb dating to 3500 B.C. It was a large bead on a necklace with a carved Turquoise ibex. Many funeral scarabs are found made of Amethyst.

Theophrastus, writing a historical treatise on gems in 300 B.C., also defined Amethyst as the "sobering gem."

In the fifteenth century, Italians used Amethyst to ward off drunkenness.

It was also written in the *Speculum Lapidum* of Camilli Leonardi (1502) that it would sober those overcome by the drunkenness of love-passion.

In Greek literature there is a city described by Lucian in his *Vera Historia* where there existed an altar made from one enormous Amethyst.

Healing Secrets

The Amethyst is a form of Quartz, a known conductor with the ability to direct waves and rays of light. The rays of life-giving Sun directed through the Amethyst crystal can effect a healing or, at the least, energize any part of the body.

Used with the light of the Moon by placing it over the heart, solar plexus, or on top of the head, it can direct the rays that control the tides to our emotional centers, putting them in balance. Because the Amethyst transmits vibrations from Mercury and Mercury especially affects all who have prominent Gemini in their natal astrology charts, it specifically works on the areas of the body ruled by Gemini—hands, arms, chest, lungs.

When lung or bronchial congestion is evident, the Amethyst has a vibration that can detect the emotional imbalance that causes this manifestation. Keep the stone as close as possible to the affected area, especially while sleeping.

The writings of Edgar Cayce contain references to the healing powers of Amethyst: "The vibration of this crystal can actually cause molecular change. In this way it can be used to heal wounds, or particularly to remove obstruction or weakness in the veins. It is also effective on broken bones."

Another psychic healer, Paul Solomon, frequently refers to Amethyst, suggesting it be worn on the chest for healing.

The Amethyst transmits cosmic rays through the "power center of communication" at the throat. The larynx and voice box contain a large group of nerves. If the words that come forth through the throat are pushed out by anger, fear, jealousy, selfishness, or any other negative emotion, their vibrations act negatively against the thyroid. This gland controls all the energies vibrating through the body.

Negative words through this power center can also cause tooth and gum disorders, sore throat, cough, and chest congestion. The tongue is closely related to the soul nature. The admonition to "watch your tongue" is one of the best possible pieces of advice.

The thyroid gland is considered by occult writers as a sex gland. Ugly words and vibrations here can cause diseases of the generative system also.

Psychic Strengths

This is a stone to be assigned for a healer. The Amethyst purifies and softens the thoughts. In order to heal others, one must be able to think in pure form. One must also perfect empathy and exercise lack of judgmental control. This stone throughout its long history has always emphasized pure, strong love. It can be used to detect ailments if the healer does not put ego ahead of the act. Even though it can be used to heal one's own ailments, all thoughts must be pure and soft before the healing takes place. Otherwise the negative acids, enzymes, and hormones continue to misbehave in the body directed by the mind.

The color vibrations in this gem suggest that an Amethyst is indicative of a creative, idealistic ability. The need to mature in judgment is present and can be fulfilled by wearing and/or carrying an Amethyst. This altruistic temperament has a tendency to take on more than it can handle. The Amethyst vibration awakens the purest analytical thinking in decisions for improving the state of the self. It also brings a higher vibration to decisions made concerning help for others. The vibration of the Amethyst for the holder will strengthen ability to express love realistically.

AMETHYST MEDITATION

The Amethyst is a stone to be assigned for a healer. It is also advised for those who wish to be a teacher, communicator, or writer.

The Amethyst vibration awakens one to purest analytical thinking in decisions for improving the state of the self. It also brings a higher vibration to decisions made concerning help for others. The vibration of the Amethyst for the holder will strengthen the ability to express love realistically.

The Amethyst, transmitting and receiving the cosmic rays of Mercury, activates the following abilities:

1. Active intelligence
2. Mind, logic, and reason
3. Educational and learning abilities
4. Spoken and written communication
5. Transmitting the spiritual to the material

Wearing the Amethyst crystal at the throat and meditating with it daily will give one the clear and pure thought of understanding and healing.

Method

Lie down on the floor on your back. Hold the Amethyst in your palm and gaze at it for one full minute.

Place the Amethyst against the . . .

SOLAR PLEXUS (near waist): Cover with palm, repeat seven times . . . "This Amethyst is vibrating to mature my judgment center."

HEART: Cover with palm, repeat seven times . . . "This Amethyst is vibrating to increase my pure healing love."

FOREHEAD ("third eye"): Cover with palm, repeat seven times . . . "This Amethyst is purifying all that comes forth in speech."

Multi-ray
Mars, Pluto, Mercury

KUNZITE

"Practitioners of all disciplines must first and foremost acquire an understanding of natural law and medicine which regards man in a holistic framework, particularly those relating to energy fields binding man and the universe."

—Dr. Wallace F. MacNaughton

▲▲▲

Both the red ray of will or power transmitted from Mars and the indigo ray of ceremonial order and control over nature from Pluto are working through the pink-lavender Kunzite. Into this interplay is added a third ray, the violet ray of Mercury, the mind.

Mars is an inner planet, while Pluto is an outer planet. Red is the first, indigo the last . . . Alpha and Omega. These are the Greek words designating the Divine Creators. This vibration, transmitted through the Kunzite, contains the

211

new promise made to Earth of unconditional love available to us through our cosmic support system.

There are three "mind power centers" (chakras) in the body that simultaneously receive these rays. The heart, genital, and sacral power centers are thinking parts of our body that have been at odds for millennia.

In our eternity of evolution we are just now beginning to understand the true meaning of the male-female life/love, desire/heart, or sex/spirit way of cohabiting Earth. Until now the primary drive has been survival as transmitted through Mars' red ray. This will, the power to live at any cost and to procreate, was the first ray.

We recall images of Neanderthal man grabbing a female by the hair and dragging her into his cave. We know that our desire body was more fully developed at that time than our soul or spirit body. According to Richard E. Leakey, the world's leading anthropologist, who continues the work of his mother and father, Louis and Mary Leakey, that scene was enacted fifty to one hundred thousand years ago.

Evolution takes a long, long time. Almost every day we read or hear about a modern-day man who has recreated Neanderthal behavior, even though he knows it constitutes a crime in our society.

The red ray from Mars must be admitted to our physical bodies to insure the continuation of life. The red-indigo ray of Pluto must be admitted to allow creation and transformation. The violet ray of Mercury, working through the "mind power center of communication," must be admitted to insure the proper balance and survival of the Mental Body. The Vital, Emotional, and Mental Bodies are all called to express and experience this Divine cooperation when Kunzite is used to transmit these cosmic rays.

This newly discovered gem is preceding the authentic ruler of its vibrations. It is transmitting from Mars, Pluto, and Mercury, but within the next several hundred years, if we can deduce from past history, a new planet will move into our solar system.

Because the Tourmaline and the Kunzite are both lithium crystals acting similarly to balance the three bodies, the planet will be close behind Vulcan. At that time, Libra will finally have its true ruler and the Zodiac will be complete.

When the pink ray is manifested, it will truly be an exalted age for Libra, the sign of marriage and partnership. In esoteric and occult literature, the pink light has always been perceived as the true light and color of love. Earth will begin to experience cooperation between nations and male-female relationships will at last come into balance.

To actually integrate the life force, the sex drive, and the spiritual love of the heart will be the next giant step in our evolution.

"We must give up our preoccupation with enemies of all kinds—we must believe that war is obsolete."

—Pierre Tielhard du Chardin

▲▲▲

KUNZITE (SPODUMENE)

CHEMICAL COMPOSITION: $LiAl(Si_2O_6)$ (lithium aluminum silicate)
CRYSTAL SYSTEM: Monoclinic
RED and VIOLET RAYS
PLANET: Mars, Pluto, and Mercury
POWER CENTER OF LOVE
POWER CENTER OF LIFE
POWER CENTER OF MIND
HEALTH FACTOR: Eyes, ears
PSYCHIC QUALITIES: Unconditional love

General Science

This spectacular lavender-pink-violet gem crystal was first described by George Frederick Kunz (1856–1932) in 1902, so it is named for him. As a world-renowned gem expert affiliated with the famous jewelry firm of Tiffany and Co., he was curator of several gem exhibitions and consultant to museums featuring outstanding gem and mineral collections.

When the Tourmaline mines were opened up in north San Diego County in the early 1900s, the companion gem crystals of Kunzite were discovered. The Pala district has the most prolific mines. The Vandenberg mine produces the best crystals for size, clarity, and coloration, while the best-formed crystals come from the Pala Chief mine nearby. The Katarina and San Pedro mines are also good producers. The Pala Chief crystals are sometimes ten inches long, which is rare.

Since the first discoveries in California at the beginning of this century, deposits have also been found in Madagascar, a large island in the Indian Ocean off the southeast coast of Africa, and in Minas Gerais, Brazil.

The faceting of Kunzite into gemstones is a tricky procedure as it has a tendency to splinter if the angle of cutting is not exactly correct. The gem has a hardness of 7 on the Mohs' scale of 1 to 10. Cut correctly, it makes a beautiful and durable gem. It does have a tendency to fade if exposed to sunlight, so it is usually styled very deeply from top to bottom to maintain as much of the lovely lilac-pink color as possible. Because it may lose color from sunlight, it is sometimes called evening stone.

Kunzite has a particular talent that it shares with the Diamond and a few other gems. It is called triboluminescence, and it is the power of storing sunlight or artificial light so that it glows. The Kunzite may do this because of manganese or uranium salts present in the crystals.

History, Myth, and Magic

Since this precious gem was so recently discovered, the research into its history has primarily been interviews with local Californians. One of the earliest natives to become totally and personally involved with Kunzite was George Ashley. He moved with his parents to the small settlement called Ramona around 1915 when he was about eleven years old. He remembers being very excited at seeing the first natural crystals of Tourmaline belonging to his playmates, who had found them in the surrounding hills. As he grew up, he recollects doing a lot of unhappy ranch work to support himself, but he was always fascinated by the crystals found in the area.

The original Kunzite discovery had been made by Frederick M. Sickler in an area of Indian grounds called Pala in north San Diego County. Sickler had sent a sample to Tiffany's in New York City, to the famous gemologist and curator G. F. Kunz, who identified it and after whom it was named. Kunz had previously identified other color deposits of this same crystal geometry as Spodumene.

Ashley remembers that around 1930 a friend of his from Encinitas, George Thompson, showed him the first faceted Kunzite he had ever seen. He said it was so astonishingly beautiful he was captivated forever. It was around this time he began learning to cut stones and to facet.

George Ashley became well-known for his gem cutting —especially Kunzite, which is very difficult, like Diamond. His continued trips to Pala to sift through the dumps of the Tourmaline mines finally led to his purchase of several small claims. In 1947 he met Frederick Sickler, who was very old and had ceased to work his two Kunzite mines, the Katarina and Vandenberg. George convinced Sickler to sell him the old house and mines. By 1950, George had found a wonderful new pocket of Kunzite and was faceting spectacular jewels that were purchased by such famous people and film stars as Lena Horne.

In 1960 the Smithsonian Institution in Washington, D.C., purchased a large collection of gem bowls and vases that George had made in his years of lapidary work. He also has another of his bowl collections on permanent display in the Museum of Natural History in Balboa Park, San Diego, California.

The accompanying mineral stone Lapidilite, which is found with Tourmaline and Kunzite, has recently been shaped into spheres and pyramids by George, one being purchased by Columbia University for its collection.

Healing Secrets

Kunzite is a lithium-bearing crystal. It is commonly known that lithium is a natural tranquilizer. In ancient Hebrew or Talmudic law, there were many admonitions concerning eating and drinking. These religious laws were originally laws of health and survival that became ritual. One such law was that no drinking water was to come from lakes or rivers. The people were instructed to dig wells and to drink only well water.

Modern scientists now comprehend that a very high percentage of underground water passes through lithium-bearing rock. Lithium is a drug that is administered to psychologically disturbed patients—especially those who are manic-depressive. It is a mood elevator and in less extreme cases is given as the tranquilizer Valium.

These lithium crystals of Kunzite are vibrating from the rays of three planets, bringing a soothing balance between the three invisible bodies of the human. The violet ray, which affects the "power center of mind," the throat chakra, is a perfect area to vibrate the Kunzite crystal.

Psychic Strengths

Lorusso and Glick, in their book *Healing Stoned*, published the therapeutic uses of gems and minerals. They devoted only three lines to Kunzite, describing it as "a stepping stone to tolerance, receptivity, and acceptance."

Richardson and Huett, in writing their book *Spiritual Value of Gem Stones*, channeled over two pages of spiritual, healing, and energy information on Kunzite. Their writings explain that Kunzite is effective in controlling erratic actions or emotions, bringing discipline, and offering a steadying influence.

In a rather large collection of books on this subject, these are the only two that give any reference to the healthful or psychic properties of Kunzite.

After carefully searching and researching, it became evident that this crystal has reached its cycle and time of discovery very close to the entry of Pluto into our solar system.

The red ray from Mars must be admitted to our physical bodies to insure the continuation of life. The red-indigo ray of Pluto must be admitted to allow creation and transformation. The violet ray of Mercury, working through the "mind power center" of communication, must be admitted to insure the proper balance and survival of the mental body. The vital body, the emotional body, and the mental body are all called to express and experience this divine cooperation when Kunzite is used to transmit these cosmic rays.

If you wish to improve the balance in your own three bodies right now, the Kunzite crystal can be used, worn on the body, carried, and held in the active meditation daily.

The special benefit of this balancing is the ability it gives to experience the unconditional love from the Universe, and to repeat that experience with all those we contact daily.

KUNZITE MEDITATION

The lithium-bearing crystals of Kunzite are vibrating the rays of three planets to bring a soothing balance between the three invisible bodies of humans. The Vital, Emotional, and Physical bodies are all called to express and experience Divine cooperation when Kunzite is used to transmit cosmic multi-rays.

Since this precious gem has been so recently discovered (1902), not much about it is known. Some experts consider it a stepping-stone to tolerance, receptivity, and acceptance. It has also been found effective in controlling erratic actions or emotions.

For those who wish to improve the balance of the three

bodies, meditation with a Kunzite crystal is suggested. The special benefit of this balancing is the ability it gives to experience unconditional love from the Universe and to repeat that experience with all those we contact.

Daily meditation with Kunzite will:

1. Bring realization of unconditional love
2. Pass this realization on to others
3. Allow healing of the three invisible bodies

Method

Lie down on the floor on your back. Hold the Kunzite in your palm and gaze at it for one full minute.

Place the Kunzite against the . . .

SOLAR PLEXUS (near waist): Cover with palm, repeat seven times . . . "This Kunzite is vibrating unconditional love from the Universe to me."

HEART: Cover with palm, repeat seven times . . . "This Kunzite is vibrating to help me pass this unconditional love on to others."

FOREHEAD ("third eye"): Cover with palm, repeat seven times . . . "This Kunzite is vibrating to allow healing of my invisible bodies."

Jupiter
The Golden Ray

TOPAZ

"All the forces of nature are constantly in flux.
A healthy person is one whose system is able
to respond quickly to change. Treatment is defined as anything which will restore balance."

—Dr. Vasant Lad
Ayurvedic Institute

▲▲▲

The golden ray-wave of the planet Jupiter enters the body through the medulla, at the base of the neck, where it activates the "mind power center of zeal." This is a very special energy that can be used to release ideas and talents, often leading to great forward steps in evolution.

Persons working with these golden ray-waves from Jupiter are always recognizable because they have remarkable energy and enthusiasm. They are true conductors of the Cosmic Current and can cheer others by the zeal they radiate. There is a passion for life and accomplishments of the spirit that are always in evidence.

Zeal is not a loud or boisterous quality. Rather, it is a magnetic, quiet vibration that attracts good positive responses of cooperation for projects and causes. When there is abuse of this zest, there may be parallel problems beginning in the neck area, where the ray enters the body. Sometimes misuse may manifest itself in needless talk and hyperactivity or meddling interference into another's beliefs.

The golden ray-waves from the planet Jupiter trigger the Higher Mind within us. Its vibrational messages include wisdom, spontaneity, optimism, enthusiasm, benevolence, the desire to gain through experience, and the wish to improve the state of things.

Jupiter's role in the cosmic family of our galaxy is twofold. Its vibration gives us confidence in the abundance of the Universe (materialism). At the same time, it elevates our minds to the philosophies of right living (spiritualism). The golden ray is, therefore, both an outgoing, beneficent ray channeling prosperity, and a retreating, inward vibration for study.

Stimulating the gold ray of Jupiter, as one would do through meditation with a Golden Topaz, will bring the wearer an increased interest in the joy of each day and a conscious awareness of the interactions of each moment. The past will fade to its proper perspective in one's memory with a renewed hope present every sunrise. It will become increasingly important to recognize that life is happening today, in the here and now. This is not a dress rehearsal. To be constantly in a state of "waiting" for the future or for a mythical "better time" is a complete denial of one's true, personal power. (Tiger's-eye also receives and transmits the golden ray. For more on it, look under the Brown Ray, it's main influence.)

Jupiter is the largest planet in our solar system, second

only to the Sun in command and influence. It represents the triumph of the spirit over the physical world. The ray-wave emanating from Jupiter helps us to be in touch with the Universal Mind and to better apply the Divine Plan to everyday living.

At this time, only the golden ray-waves from Jupiter and the green rays of Saturn can be identified as being transmitted by the gem Peridot. This gem crystal seems to affect Librans. (For more on Peridot, look under its main planet, Saturn.)

Astrology gives Libra the rule of the human anatomy governing the kidney area. In her writing from Charles Fillmore's theories on the twelve power centers of the body, Catherine Ponder, in *The Healing Secret of the Ages,* calls this area the "mind power center of elimination."

Every major function of the physical body corresponds to an invisible Emotional, Mental, and Spiritual body within us. Elimination is a physical function that screens and drains off all unnecessary poisons and bulk from our physical system. It also rids the mind, emotions, and spirit of poison.

Possessiveness is poison. We must learn to eliminate holding on to another person as if we owned them. By acknowledging that all things are borrowed from an abundant Universe, we can relieve our mental grasping.

The Peridot is a double light refractor, bringing twice the pressure to focus on the elimination of possessiveness in our lives. Eliminating negative emotions, beliefs, and habits of spirit is the quickest way to freedom. Giving up the poison and bulk that we have accumulated is such a relief that the body actually becomes lighter.

We cannot take anything with us when we leave this Earth. Therefore, we do not own anything nor anyone. Even our soul belongs to the Universal Spirit.

Elimination also occurs as a function of the skin and lungs. The skin perspires to eliminate excess moisture, and we expel used air from the lungs. Physical exercise is a natural way to rid the poisons and bulk from the body.

Peridot is also transmitting the ray-waves of a still unseen planet, soon to be the ruler of Libra. The history of metaphysics has shown change is felt before it actually occurs.

Libra is depicted as balance. It is an intellectual and communicative air sign meant to express its outgoing, initiatory, cardinal nature harmoniously. These positive traits cannot be expressed if the "mind power center of elimination" is backed up with refuse.

Possessive emotions, insistence upon holding on to old and outworn crystallized belief systems, or grasping for material goods are all symptoms that the Peridot is needed to aid in elimination.

The fact that certain types of meteors falling to Earth contain Peridot (Olivine) tells us that somewhere in outer space there is a planet sending physical transmitters to precede itself. We will use this gift wisely if we cleanse ourselves by getting rid of all disbelief and opening to new thought in a New Age.

TOPAZ

CHEMICAL COMPOSITION: $Al_2(OH,F)(SiO_4)$ (neosilicate ion)
CRYSTAL SYSTEM: Orthorhombic
RAY: Yellow
PLANET: Jupiter
POWER CENTER OF ZEAL
HEALTH FACTOR: Pituitary, vitamin-hormone balance
PSYCHIC QUALITIES: Joy, living in the moment, optimism

General Science

The name derives from the Greek island of Topazos. This name was formerly applied to some gemstone whose identity has been lost, but whose coloring was similar to the presently named gem.

The crystals occur generally in stubby to medium-long diamond shapes. Crystals range in size from very small to some of several hundred pounds in weight. Usually the faces of prisms are present. The crystals are transparent to translucent. Often the coloring is similar to Aquamarine, or brownish orange. The color that we are dealing with here, that is most commonly known and accepted, is yellow-gold. On a scale of 1 to 10, it has a hardness of 8. The color is produced by the elements aluminum hydroxyl-fluorine silicate. The steady movement of electrons or electrical current occurs only in crystals with a metallic bond. The aluminum bond gives Topaz this power.

Topaz is found in many areas on Earth, namely California, Colorado, Utah, Nigeria, West Africa, Burma, Germany, Ireland, Japan, and Australia. The very finest specimens are found in Russia, with the next best gems in quality and size found in Brazil. Light blue Topaz are also found in Ireland, Scotland, and Cornwall, England.

There are many yellow or gold-colored stones that may be confused with Topaz. Some Mexican Amethysts can be heat-treated to look like Topaz. Smokey Quartz is often mistaken for Smokey Topaz. Citrine is also used for Topaz, but has a lower hardness, as it is a Quartz variety also. The crystal formation of Topaz is completely different in geometry from Quartz. Yellow Beryl or Aquamarine, yellow Rubies or Sapphires, Spinel and Tourmaline, may be confused with Topaz.

Mining Topaz is a slow, manual process. Authentic Topaz is more rare and more expensive in the yellow colors due to its smaller availability in the market. The golden natural Topaz of this treatise is called Precious Topaz. This is only found in veins formed by fluorine gas escaping from cooling magma.

Light blue Topaz is more common and is now being used in place of Aquamarine as good, clear Beryl is so scarce.

History, Myth, and Magic

The oldest Chinese writings refer to the Topaz as one of five stones to be made into an amulet and placed at the entrance of one's home to draw the planetary rays that would protect and enhance the family living there.

The Smithsonian Institution in Washington, D.C., has a most extensive gem and mineral collection. It has faceted Topaz on display of several thousand carats. In 1965, in the Russian Ukraine, a Blue Topaz of 220 pounds was reportedly mined. In Portugal, the crown contains a clear Topaz that was thought to be a Diamond for many years. It is a famous stone called the Braganza. It weighs over one thousand carats.

An exceptional Topaz crystal, three inches in diameter and two inches high, was pictured on the cover of *Lapidary Journal* in August 1981. Amazingly, the crystal was collected in 1875 from Siberia, USSR, and has been protected from light for over a century. It is in the University of Paris collection. The wife of curator D. Pierre Bariande, Nellie Bariande, has photographed it very carefully by long exposure in subdued light. Light would cause this Topaz to turn blue. This is the only known photograph of an orange Siberian Topaz.

Healing Secrets

The Topaz vibration is soft, steady, and expansively giving. This vibration is helpful to combat insomnia. In the same way, it will relieve a tension headache. If you are a healer, the yellow Topaz is excellent for use with warm light, either Sun or incandescent, passing through onto the affected area of the body. This is called pyroelectricity, or the stimulation of the electrons in the crystal. This in turn causes the blood vessels to expand, allowing greater circulation. Increased circulation brings more oxygen to the brain. Deep breathing will also give this effect, so combining the two is twice as helpful. The resulting feeling is one of mellowness and well-being.

Fluorine is a rare element found in Topaz. You will discover in healing with a Topaz that the preservation of calcium in the body will be improved.

The Topaz, in responding to the ray-waves of the planet Jupiter, would be astrologically formulated to affect the hips and thighs. Since one of the most common problems of people over seventy is a broken hip or disintegration of the hip joint, osteoporosis, the fluorine vibration could very well strengthen the calcium skeletal part of the hips and thighs. As a preventive, it would be worn on the body at all times. As a healing aid, it would be placed on the bony area anywhere on the body in direct sunlight or a suitable substitute.

Psychic Strengths

The basic psychic vibration of the Topaz is hope. It is optimism and a belief in a good future. If a Topaz is recommended or chosen, it is an indication that negative thoughts, and a feeling of fear, need to be replaced.

Bringing up the vibration of the spirit also brings up the

vibration of the body. Fear of failure is very destructive to many areas of the body. It causes the muscles in the neck and shoulders to contract. This affects the pineal gland, which consequently sets off the body's alarm system, which if overused, will ultimately destroy both bone and muscle cartilage. The Topaz has a quieting, mellowing effect on this psychic fear.

Choosing Topaz is also an indication that not enough emphasis is being given to living in the present moment. A conscious effort must be exerted by the holder to concentrate on being more fully aware of each moment. The joy and beauty of life can be realized if we live as though there were not a tomorrow. The Topaz is a reminder to release *all* of the past and not wait for tomorrow—but to live fully today.

TOPAZ MEDITATION

The vibration of the Topaz is hope. It offers optimistic belief in a good future that will replace negative thoughts and fears.

The soft, steady Topaz vibration is helpful against insomnia. Used in meditation, it establishes a mellow sense of well-being that also relieves tension headaches.

Fluorine is a rare element within the Topaz that preserves and improves the calcium in the body. In responding to the ray-waves of Jupiter, which by astrological formula affects the hips and thigh, Topaz offers a remedy to strengthen these areas that are often disabled through osteoporosis.

Meditation with Topaz will raise the vibration of the

spirit while at the same time raising the vibration of the body. It will:

1. Bring joy and hope back into the consciousness
2. Relieve negative thoughts and fear
3. Demand that full attention be given to living NOW
4. Relieve muscle tenseness, which inhibits Cosmic Consciousness and destroys the joints in the body

Method

Lie down on the floor on your back. Hold the Topaz in your palm and gaze at it for one full minute.

Place the Topaz against the . . .

SOLAR PLEXUS (near waist): Cover with palm, repeat seven times . . . "This Topaz is vibrating to restore my joy and hope."

HEART: Cover with palm, repeat seven times . . . "This Topaz is vibrating to relieve my negative thoughts and fears."

FOREHEAD ("third eye"): Cover with palm, repeat seven times . . . "This Topaz is vibrating to focus my attention to living NOW."

The Brown Ray
Jupiter and
Unknown Source

TIGER'S-EYE

"The will is my real self. The body is my expression of the will."

—Arthur Schopenhauer

▲▲▲

The Tiger's-eye receives and transmits the golden cosmic ray from Jupiter and the brown ray from an undiscovered source.

In James Sturzaker's work *The Twelve Rays*, he extends the seven rays of Alice Bailey's *Treatise on the Seven Rays* to twelve, including the brown ray, a mixture of indigo and orange. He actualizes the vibration of the brown ray as study, concentration, and absorption of knowledge. Higher levels of the gold and brown ray represent wisdom.

One of the admired sects of devotion in the Christian organization, the Franciscan monks, reflects the brown ray in their brown, hooded robes. Their consciousness and focus are total concentration in truth.

The brown ray vibration quiets the "mind chatter" that is so distracting to soul evolution. When this quieting takes place, the mind opens for higher work. Often there is an increase in silent communication abilities. Clairvoyance or telepathic connections are frequently the outcome.

The vibration of the gem-ray connection between Tiger's-eye, the unknown planet (brown ray), and Jupiter's golden ray of higher mind and intellect strengthens the will. Arthur Schopenhauer, the German metaphysical philosopher (1788–1860) expressed the relationship of will to the material: "The will is my real self. The body is my expression of the will."

Strengthening the will means finding the balance between intuition and willfulness. To use the power of will to enhance the quality of life is to consciously decide when one's imagination is needed, or when determination is the answer.

Unbridled willfulness causes tension to mount in the body, especially in the head. This is due to the concentration of mind power in the forehead, which, if unchecked, results in constriction of the blood vessels, causing acute headache. There is a difference, of course, between willfulness and willpower. The power of the will to focus and concentrate on right actions must be balanced with self-love and the love of others.

TIGER'S-EYE

(Quartz Group)
CHEMICAL COMPOSITION: SiO_2 (silicone dioxide)
CRYSTAL SYSTEM: Hexagonal (trigonal)
BROWN and YELLOW RAYS
PLANET: Jupiter
POWER CENTER OF WILL
HEALTH FACTOR: Medulla (brain), headache relief
PSYCHIC QUALITIES: Concentration, focusing energy

General Science

The name of this stone comes from its appearance and coloring. It is a type of stone referred to as "chatoyant," derived from a French verb meaning "to gleam like the eyes of a cat." The bright, brownish-yellow streaks of the Tiger's-eye are caused when Quartz flows into a cavity and traps iron and asbestos particles within. This combination makes an opaque stone with a pearlized silky reflection of gold to brown.

There are two other stones of the same Quartz base that have slightly different elements. One is the Quartz Cat's-eye, which is almost pearly white. The other is the Hawk's-eye, colored in blue-grays. In all the Quartz varieties, the hardness on a scale of 1 to 10 is 7.

The most important deposits of Tiger's-eye are found in South Africa. Other deposits are located in Australia, Burma, India, Mexico, and California.

History, Myth, and Magic

One of the earliest uses of the Tiger's-eye, also known at times as Chalcedony, was for production of amulets in an

Assyrio-Babylonian era. These were cut in cylinders, covered with carved figures and symbols, and pierced at one end. There are examples in famous world museums dating from 4000 B.C. Scholars disagree about their uses. Some contend they were simply signature seals used with wax or ink, while others feel they were worn around the neck for protection. Possibly they were used for both purposes. Their designs often represent religious or mythical figures and the written names of gods.

An old Spanish list, translated from Arabic in 1604, names the Tiger's-eye as the stone corresponding to Capricorn in the zodiac. Capricorn is ruled by Saturn, and Saturn is considered the strict schoolmaster of the Universe. This celestial teacher insists that we do our homework. In this translation, the Tiger's-eye represents the focus of energy on learning.

Thesaurus Philosophicus Seu de Gemmis, written in 1702 by Josehpi Gonelli, states that the Tiger's-eye would drive away ghosts and phantoms of the night. Due to the fact that cats can see in the dark, the stone was also said to improve the night vision of its owner.

Healing Secrets

The vibrations of the Tiger's-eye have an especially helpful healing effect on the muscles surrounding the upper neck and scalp. These muscles tend to constrict when a person is charged with a superkinetic energy. This energy, if not directed toward a constructive outlet, turns in upon itself and puts tension on various muscles. Another area of tension is in the muscles around the knees. In both areas, this muscle tension causes constriction of blood vessels. When the natural flow of circulation is tampered with, pain is the ultimate result. Headache and neckache are common.

Muscle constriction in the head is often severe around

the eyes and will cause the vision to be affected. One of the first signs of an approaching "migraine" headache is a vision change, signaled by either spots or a white light in the peripheral range. If this is a constant area of constriction, there will eventually be permanent damage to the eye muscles.

Similarly, the muscles in the knees and neck can restrict the flow of blood in those areas, until the bone and cartilage are actually broken down and pain becomes constant. Since it is the mind that sends the signals to the muscles, it is then imperative for the mind to work on accepting the soothing vibration of the Tiger's-eye. The rhythm of this particular vibration should be allowed to become a song that invades the innermost recesses of thought and soothes the frantic jumble of notes that are not harmonious. This will noticeably slow down the energy. When this energy becomes more regulated, it can focus on fewer objects outside the body. It is important to direct the focus away from the *constriction* of our own muscles and into the *construction* of some useful property, both for ourselves and others.

This superkinetic energy is a wonderful gift often born with highly evolved individuals. If this energy is not focused, it will spray out uncontrollably, sometimes being harmful, not only to the body of the individual but also to other sensitive people with whom they come in contact. Most often close relatives or mates are affected. Casual acquaintances may also feel the agitation or uncomfortable effects of this energy. Not knowing what it is, they may back away.

As the individual is able to meditate and integrates the focusing vibrations of the Tiger's-eye into their own, the calming effect will become noticeable. Nervousness and uncontrolled thoughts drop away. Their schedule becomes less overcrowded; more projects are completed. The energy is at last focused, harnessed, and directed.

Psychic Strengths

The Tiger's-eye vibration is very regulated and precise, like a metronome or ticking clock. It is a vibration that goes in and out, however, not back and forth. The pumping of the heart is expanding and contracting like the vibration of the Tiger's-eye . . . reaching out . . . pulling in. As a regulator, its basic message is to bring back to center the scattered energy. In so doing it opens up the action of the solar plexus, the center of being. This area is in the centripetal center of our body, the seat of our emotions or feelings. It is the area affected when we perceive danger or sexual excitement. We feel "butterflies," or a fluttering motion there, sometimes like an upward motion moving in the direction of our heart. When we become more "centered" by using the Tiger's-eye in meditation, the solar plexus develops beyond the primal feeling stage of fear and excitement into a more advanced stage of feeling the thoughts and actions of others. We can become much more psychic in our communication with others around us.

By centering our energies we increase the power of our solar plexus to search out with invisible probes the person or group that will be compatible, sympathetic, or supportive of our projects, motives, and desires. The opening up on the solar plexus area is also a freeing experience. When this most important part of ourselves has been starved and neglected, it becomes weak and unable to function. It is like a prisoner in solitary confinement existing on bread and water, still alive, but operating only in a state of survival. In this state it cannot give us the pleasure it was designed to give. We lose our capacity to *feel* deeply. The first thing we lose is the feeling of true love.

As the meditation becomes an automatic part of our daily routine, our energies begin to come together in the center of our being. The first signs of this will be a slowing down of the body activity. There will be greater periods of physical inactivity. In these times, our personal vibrations are beginning to integrate with the Tiger's-eye vibrations. It is a natural reaction to feel some discomfort about this, even guilt. Depending on how many years we have been operating in a "hyperkinetic" state, we will feel symptoms that are very similar to withdrawal from drugs or alcohol.

This hyperkinetic energy is often overlooked in the young, who as children are regarded by many as bratty, willful, spoiled, and aggravating. In young adults it is laughed off as rambunctious energy, "sowing wild oats," immaturity, or the inability to live up to potential. This begins to take a negative turn somewhere around the age of thirty. By the time a man reaches thirty-five or a woman reaches forty, they are beginning to get some inkling of the fact that their "potential" is not materializing. At this time, there is a tendency to become frequently despondent and to accept failure, in fact, to court failure by increasing activity. This is a frantic flailing about to *do* something to alleviate the stress, or to *do* something to bring about success. The only formula that works is the one most overlooked. As the teacher Jesus told us, "It is so simple, it confounds the wise." To go within ourselves, to quiet the body, quiet the mind, and let the spirit speak to us seems so simple.

When we free our emotional self, it can operate with all its many talents, to signal us when we are on the track or off. Gradually it begins to repay us for its freedom with the feeling that we have missed for so long, the feeling of love.

TIGER'S-EYE MEDITATION

The vibrations of the Tiger's-eye have an especially helpful healing effect on the muscles surrounding the upper neck and scalp. These muscles tend to constrict when an individual is charged with a superkinetic energy, which if undirected, turns in upon itself, putting tension on various muscles.

Depending on how many years an individual has been operating in a hyperkinetic state, they will experience symptoms very similar to a withdrawal from drugs or alcohol.

If you are doing a lot but not getting anything done, hooked on activity but not acting in your own best interests, meditate daily with the Tiger's-eye in order to focus your mind to:
1. Slow down the personal vibration
2. Focus your energy
3. Relieve nervous time-wasting
4. Regulate eating habits

Method

Lie down on the floor on your back. Hold the Tiger's-eye in your palm and gaze at it for one full minute.

Place the Tiger's-eye against the . . .
SOLAR PLEXUS (near waist): Cover with palm, repeat seven times . . . "This Tiger's-eye is vibrating to pull back all my scattered energy into the center of myself."
HEART: Cover with palm, repeat seven times . . . "This Tiger's-eye is vibrating so that I may be quiet to feel love again."
FOREHEAD ("third eye"): Cover with palm, repeat seven times . . . "This Tiger's-eye is vibrating to focus my mind energy for my own benefit and the service of others."

Multi-ray
Vulcan
The Hidden Planet

TOURMALINE

"The other prevailing hypothesis supports the long recognized possibility that the sun has a small but faithful companion, with a mass of about 7% of that of the sun. This sister star exists either in the visible or the invisible (infrared) parts of the light spectrum."

—*Science News,* Vol. 125
May 1984

▲▲▲

The multi-ray of Vulcan, transmitting through Tourmaline, is entering our body's judgment center to put the Mental and Spiritual Body into balance with the physical body. Whoever uses the Tourmaline must be prepared for the transformation of the three bodies.

The Tourmaline, with its pleochroism (reflection of three different rays or angles of light), is the youngest historical gem to surface in enough quantity and quality worldwide actually to affect a balancing of these three bodies.

Discoveries of Tourmaline in Afghanistan will have a burning effect on the Middle East for some years to come, personally and historically. The strength of this gem will "set fire" to the places of judgment in the body, often causing the sensation of heat.

In burning old judgments and giving up the mind-set that causes certain ailments, there will be inner struggles painfully taking place in the emotional psyche. This will mean a personal dedication to undergo heat and pressure in order to balance the trinity within.

Vulcan is already stimulating health-minded individuals worldwide to concentrate on holistic centers to raise consciousness. We humans are designed to live longer, to accomplish more, and to be happy. Tourmaline and Vulcan are working together for a new age of vital living.

TOURMALINE

CHEMICAL COMPOSITION: $(NaLiCa)(Fe_{11}Mg\ Mn\ Pl)_3AL_6(OH)_4(Bo_3)Si_6O_{18})$ (aluminum borate) (Silicate, complicated and changeable composition. Double light refraction.)

CRYSTAL SYSTEM: Hexagonal (trigonal)

MULTI-RAY

PLANET: Vulcan (Yet unseen)

POWER CENTER OF ORDER

HEALTH FACTORS: Intestinal tract

PSYCHIC QUALITIES: Balances the Physical, Mental, Emotional, and Spiritual bodies

General Science

The Tourmaline has more variation and richness of color than any other gem. According to color, there are seven varieties:

Acroite—Greek for colorless. Rare.

Rebellite—Latin for red or pink (ruby color most valuable).

Dravite—Austrian for yellow brown to dark brown.

Verdelite—Latin-Greek for green in all shades (emerald green the best).

Indigolite—blue in all shades.

Siberite—Russian, lilac to violet.

Schorl—black, very common, old mining term (rarely used for jewelry).

On the Mohs' scale for hardness of 1 to 10, Tourmaline measures 7. Because of its color abundance, Tourmaline may be mistaken for Amethyst, Emerald, Ruby, Citrine, and many other stones. Certain identification would be the high double refraction of light and trichromism (where three colors can be detected).

Colorless Tourmaline is very rare. The South African stones are interestingly called watermelon because they are colored pink inside and green outside. The Brazilian stones provide an even more perfect example of watermelon shading as they also include the white part of the green rind, found next to the pink. These are best seen in a cross-section slice of crystal.

Tourmaline crystals grow in very slender, elongated shapes, similar to Emerald and Aquamarine beryl. Its hexagonal lineage makes it a cousin to both beryl and Quartz, and it shares the interior trigonal geometry with Amethyst.

The most productive deposits are found in Brazil, Sri Lanka, and the Malagasy Republic. Further deposits are found in Switzerland, Russia, Thailand, Tanzania, Namibia, Zimbabwe, India, Burma, Australia, Angola, and North America. There are several states—Colorado, Connecticut, New York, Maine, and California—where mining takes place.

History, Myth, and Magic

Although there is some written history of the gem dating from antiquity, it was not until 1703 that the Tourmaline was brought to the Western world. Dutch traders imported the gem from Sri Lanka, then known as Ceylon. The gem was called Turamali, a Sinhalese name that cannot be translated.

The Dutch learned of the magnetic properties of the stone. By heating and cooling, or rubbing with pressure, a Tourmaline crystal will become electrically charged. One end becomes negative, the other positive. They put this to good Dutch practical use. A heated crystal would magnetize and pull the ashes out of their meerschaum pipes. For many years the gem was called Aschentrekker, which means "ash-puller" in German.

A book published in the United States by the California State Division of Mines, *Minerals of California*, proves that the American Indians valued and used the crystals long before white men knew anything about them.

Historical reports give credit to Henry Hamilton, who first discovered gem Tourmalines in Riverside County in 1872. There were doubtless other mines and miners, but at that time they kept their finds a secret. The recorded lists of California minerals did not contain Tourmaline until some years later. In 1895, Charles Russell Orcut, a botanist-scientist, on a field trip, discovered a large deposit of pink Tourmaline near Temecula, in north San Diego County. In 1902, several discoveries at Pala and Mesa Grande attracted attention. The Great Pala Chief mine and Himalaya mines, found in 1903, have yielded the most spectacular specimens.

The Boxer Rebellion around 1900 ended the shipments to China of Tourmaline for carving. This rebellion may in fact have been precipitated by the actual influences of the message-vibrations of the gem. "Boxer" is a translation of a Chinese phrase that means "righteous uniting band." The Boxer Rebellion against foreign powers and foreigners in China was unsuccessful.

On the surface it appeared that China was actually set back in its progress. Metaphysically speaking, however, this merely lent courage to the Chinese people, who later joined Mao Tse-tung. They revolted completely against the old and devastating order of the elite monarchy, overthrowing the stifling ways of serfdom. Tourmaline sculptures still grace the hidden places of luxury enjoyed by the political rulers of the revolutionized, communist China.

Healing Secrets

This gem is conducting the ray-waves of the yet unseen planet Vulcan. The portion of the human body that is affected and ruled by these vibrations is located in the solar plexus. The specific area is the stomach, however, all the digestive tract is included. The liver, gall bladder, and pancreas are involved.

Whether the gem is used by a healer or the afflicted person uses it on himself, the placement of the stone against the solar plexus will direct the ray-waves. The addition of sunlight, or artificial light, will aid the process. The three-way light refraction of this gem is the unusual secret of its strength.

Psychic Strengths

The judgment center of the mental body resides in the solar plexus. The analytical left brain is also involved in judgment. The planet Vulcan represents "transformation by fire and pressure." The mystical and metaphysical symbolism of fire is "purification."

The judgment centers are very life-giving, saving, and protecting for the human, both mentally and physically as well as spiritually. The message of a life choosing to work with Tourmaline helps the soul understand Health (Body), Work (Mind), and Service (Spirit).

The action of fire is considered negative by the uninitiated. In occult knowledge, it provides insight and is a natural promoter of growth . . . ask any farmer who burns the chaff in his fields. The purification by fire is both literal and figurative.

The practice of medicine, surgery, repair and healing, has made tremendous strides in this century alone. Unfortunately we have managed to keep a certain percentage of ourselves in sickness and disease. But we are recognizing that mental and spiritual disorder create illness where there is no structural inclination.

TOURMALINE MEDITATION

The portion of the human body that is affected and ruled by the vibrations of the unseen planet, Vulcan, is located in the solar plexus.

Whether the gem is used by a healer upon another, or if the sufferers use it on themselves, the placement of the stone against the solar plexus will direct the ray-waves.

The addition of sunlight, or artificial light, will definitely assist the process. The three-way light refraction of this gem is the unusual secret of its strength.

Tourmaline, only now beginning its glorious ascent to recognition, will affect and inspire those who come in contact with it in the future, particularly those working in the areas of health and humanitarian service. Meditation with this stone will:

1. Transform harsh judgment to wisdom
2. Balance logic and intuition
3. Align the physical, mental, emotional, and spiritual bodies
4. Heal the stomach and digestive system

Method

Lie down on the floor on your back. Hold the Tourmaline in your palm and gaze at it for one full minute.

Place the Tourmaline against the . . .

SOLAR PLEXUS (near waist): Cover with palm, repeat seven times . . . "This Tourmaline is vibrating to transform my judgment center."

HEART: Cover with palm, repeat seven times . . . "This Tourmaline is vibrating to increase my intuition."

FOREHEAD ("third eye"): Cover with palm, repeat seven times . . . "This Tourmaline is vibrating to align my physical, mental, emotional, and spiritual bodies."

Ultraviolet Ray
Neptune
OPAL

The Opal is a transmitter for the planet Neptune, whose vibrations reach us on an ultraviolet ray-wave, entering the body through the pineal gland within our brain. The human eye has not developed, as yet, an ability to see the ultraviolet in our spectrum.

The planet of Neptune is mysterious to us because it is so very far away. Astrologers believe that Neptune, first sighted in our solar system in 1846, is not really a member of our solar system at all, but is functioning as a transmitter of "galactic energies" to our system.

Neptune is seen as a planet of feminine influence, even though it is represented by a masculine god. In mythology,

King Neptune was known as the ruler of the seas. The feminine influences attributed to the vibrational ray-waves of the planet are: impressionable, sensitive, reflective, fluidic, and receptive. All these adjectives can also be applied to bodies of water.

The greatest mysteries still unexplained to us on Earth remain in our oceans. Even though we are nurtured in amniotic fluid for the nine months prior to birth, many of us are never comfortable going underwater during our lifetime.

The amorphous Opal is the only precious gem that contains such a high percentage of water. Its unusual structure eluded scientific description until late in this century. Transmitting Neptunian ray-waves, the Opal works on unconscious and subconscious levels.

Positive Neptunian attributes include spirituality, intuition, inspiration, and clairvoyance. In the negative, they are seen as delusions, chaotic mental conditions, incoherence, and deception.

The Opal and Neptune, working through the "mind power center of understanding," enable us to receive knowledge from sources above reason. When one has worked many lifetimes on the center of understanding, their present incarnation will be in cycle and timing to merge the mind with superphysical beings. This is known in psychic circles as channeling information from a higher source.

Neptune entered Capricorn, the tenth sign of the zodiac, on January 8, 1984, where it will remain (except for its brief trip back into Sagittarius in 1984) until 1998. During this fourteen year period, the nebulous planet will affect the world's business consciousness.

We will see an increase in psychic abilities, clairvoyance, telepathy, and possibly a blending of art and music for healing. There will be an increase in businesses dealing with the occult mystical and metaphysical aspects of life, with significant advances in medicine and healing brought forth by scientists "tuned in" to superphysical beings who will inspire them.

Keep in mind that Neptune's influence is a very subtle vibration. These things will not burst upon us, but will be developed in our subconscious "mind power center of understanding."

At the same time, those who have not prepared for this time will respond to the negative possibilities. Drug abuse, alcoholism, depression, and delusions are the most common forms manifested by the unprepared.

Those individuals who are ready for the use of the Opal and the ultraviolet ray-waves of Neptune will be compelled to act as instruments for the advancement of the superphysical understanding of mankind.

The Opal transmits the Silver ray from the Moon also. The Moon controls the fluid of the Earth and its inhabitants as well. Since the Opal has such a high percentage of water within its structure, it is a very good example of the effects of the Moon on human psyche.

For more information on these qualities, see the description of the Silver ray.

OPAL

(Quartz Group)
CHEMICAL COMPOSITION: $SiO_2 \cdot nH_2O$ (hydrous silicon dioxide)
CRYSTAL SYSTEM: Generally called amorphous, having no definite composition. Recently technology has shown that Opals are composed of tiny spheres containing very minute crystals of crytobalite mineral layered in jelly. In many instances Opals contain up to thirty percent water.
ULTRAVIOLET RAYS (Also silver and white rays)
PLANET: Neptune
POWER CENTER OF UNDERSTANDING
HEALTH FACTORS: Feet
PSYCHIC QUALITIES: Left brain, psychic awareness

General Science

The special characteristic of the Opal is a rainbowlike iridescence, changing with the angle of light that enters. It is found in three basic background colors, milky white, dark gray/black, or red. The red Opals very seldom contain rainbow opalescence. Since the stone contains a lot of moisture, its beauty will be preserved if it is stored in damp wool. Heat can dry out the Opal and cause it to crack. Jewelers need to be reminded that to be more protective and to increase the lasting beauty of the stone, mountings should be built slightly higher than the stone. As its beauty is especially enhanced by cutting and polishing "en cabochon" (a smooth domed shape), it is vulnerable to scratches and knocks. On a hardness scale of 1 to 10, the Opal rates 5½–6. Its softness is greater than most stones mounted in cabochon shape, which warrants the extra care. Acids and alkalies also affect the Opal. It should be removed from the body if soaps or lotions containing these chemicals are used.

Opal is not a product of melting or heat, the source of formation of many gems in igneous rock. Although classified in the Quartz group because of the high silicon content, it is much lighter, contains many pores, and does not grow in crystals. It is formed by evaporation. The original "seed" may be a minute group of crystals, but the whole product is not crystalline in structure. This very fact gives it a mysterious quality and sets it apart from all other gems. There are more than 150 terms used to describe various Opal varietes, including Wood Opal, Moss Opal, Hydrophane, Hyalite, Cachalong, and others, but only the three mentioned by color—milky white, dark gray/black, and red—are considered precious.

Before 1900 the best Opals were found in Czechoslovakia. Deposits were discovered in Australia and are currently the best known sources. Small deposits have been found in the United States, the best located in Nevada, with others in Idaho, Washington, and Oregon. Other mines are operating in Brazil, Guatemala, Honduras, and Japan. The important Fire Opal is mined principally in Mexico.

The market is full of Opals that have been tampered with to enhance their appearance or have been manufactured synthetically. Some are dyed black, and others are glued to a backing with black glue. Some white Opals are actually "doublets," a thin slice of precious Opal glued to common Opal. "Triplets" are the same with a layer of rock crystal added to the top. Synthetic Opals are now produced and intermixed with others on the market. Be sure you buy from a reputable, knowledgeable dealer.

History, Myth, and Magic

The modern name "Opal" is derived from three ancient sources. The oldest is the Sanskrit "upala." The Latin is "opalus," and the Greek, "ophthalmos."

The earliest written accounts of the Opal appear very late in history compared with references to other gems. There is no mention of Opal in biblical or rabbinical texts. Although the word "upala" is found in Sanskrit, the oldest written language, neither the Hindu religion or early astrological writings make any reference to it, at least in descriptions we can recognize today.

The first account is included in the *Natural History* of Pliny the Elder, written between A.D. 23 and 79. His text went into more detail about Opal than any other gem. He wrote about a large Opal owned by Senator Nonious. Mark Anthony saw the Opal and wanted to give it to Cleopatra. Nonious refused to part with it and because of his attachment to the Opal, was forced to flee Rome and Mark Anthony's anger. He left all of his possessions, except the Opal. Much later, in the 1700s, an Opal was unearthed during excavation work in Alexandria in Egypt. It was set in a ring exactly as had been described by Pliny seventeen centuries earlier.

The Opal has been the victim of dichotomies since the 1600s, with much contradiction as to whether it was good or evil. The English spelling at that time was *Ophal*, derived from *ophthalmos*, meaning "pertaining to the eye." Older myths from Scandinavia told of the god Vulcan making Opals from the eyes of children, which created a gruesome reputation for the gem.

There were many superstitions about the fearsome "evil eye." But contrary reports claimed the Opal had a very good effect on the eye itself, benefiting sight. Others reported an opposite power. For instance, Agricola wrote in *De Natura Fossilum* in 1546 that the Opal had the power to render the owner invisible to other's eyes. This is actually true when we consider the ability of the mental body to travel through extrasensory perception (ESP) without the physical body.

The Opal suffered a short period of disfavor due to a

popular book written by Sir Walter Scott in the mid-1800s in which the doomed heroine wore Opal combs in her hair. It then returned to favor when Queen Victoria, a most important person historically, made the Opal popular by giving one to each of her daughters on their wedding days.

The fact that the Opal's reputation for centuries has varied from blessing to disruption is completely valid. It depends entirely upon the hand in which it is held. Today there are many who are spiritually evolved enough to use the Opal; there are others who will be distressed or made nervous by the gem. The extra information that flows into the senses when the Opal is used can aid metaphysicians, counselors, healers, and the secular world of politicians, arbitrators, and counselors of law. These persons are directly responsible for the communication that will aid the world's nations in understanding each other.

The first reference to the Opal surfaced around 1450, coincident with the life of the great astronomer Copernicus, who revolutionized world thought regarding the relationship of the Earth to the Universe.

Leonardo da Vinci was one of our modern-day prophets, astounding his contemporaries and us to this day with wild imaginings of machinery and contraptions to fly man about. He was a painter, sculptor, architect, engineer, and scientist of the highest order. Is it any wonder or coincidence that Italian and Polish lists of birthstones named the Opal during da Vinci's lifetime (1452–1519)?

All these giant steps for mankind were not mere coincidence. There is a blueprint for our existence. What we find within the Earth corresponds to what we find on the Earth's surface and what we will find in the heavens.

There is a current influx of Opal, being distributed worldwide for the first time. The Australian finds of precious Opal have sparked a commercial interest that is not to be taken lightly. The amazing thing concerning this discovery is that it occurred in an area inhabited for 16,000 years by a very able and mystical race of aborigines, one of the four recognized races of people on Earth, called Australoid. Their culture appears on the surface to be very primitive. It was this mistaken idea that caused the Europeans, who invaded their homeland when America was having its revolution, to unmercifully commit genocide on the aborigine population. Since 1780 their numbers have dwindled from 300,000 (500 tribes) to 80,000 half- and full-blooded aborigines. The Europeans found a people who lived in peace. They were neither competitive nor violent. They had a very complex society with 700 different languages, used for various rituals or aspects of communication.

Anthropological studies that have taken place in the last one hundred years have uncovered amazing abilities among these people in the areas of telepathy and extrasensory perception, which is practiced by them as an everyday occurrence, as normal as speaking. For 16,000 years they have been walking, sleeping, and hunting over fields of Opals.

Healing Secrets

"From head to toe" is a very common phrase. It particularly suits the Opal with regard to the healing process. The planet Neptune transmits through the pineal gland in the head and also rules the feet. In the modern healing processes there is much emphasis put on the aspect of touching. Many clinical tests have shown that homo sapiens are very much like the animal kingdom . . . we need petting and stroking. Physical therapy, therapeutic massage, acupuncture, acupressure, and reflexology are showing marvelous results in improving the state of health.

Reflexology deals with the nerve endings and pressure points on the soles of the feet (and palms) that correspond to all parts of the body. Any area of the body can be treated by massaging and applying pressure to the sole at the proper point. The Opal, transmitting Neptune's ray-waves, would be of great benefit to slide over the soles during this treatment. In cases of actual deformity or pain in the feet, the Opal working with the ray-waves of Neptune can offer relief. When soaking the feet, drop an Opal into the water and notice the vibrational change.

The physical makeup of an Opal corresponds to the physical properties of the brain. Although the brain has been studied constantly with tools developed through our expanded technology of the last century, it still remains a mystery to us. The Opal is much the same. The colors perceived are almost pure spectrum colors, resulting from a narrow band of wavelengths that are very special. There are many waves in what we call light. In the Opal, and only in the Opal, are found the waves not destroyed by interference after reflection from thin films within the stone.

We know that waves emanate from the brain. We know that the brain receives sensory impulses and transmits motor impulses. It is composed of gray matter (the outer cortex of nerve cells), and white matter (inner mass of nerve fibers). This corresponds to black Opals and white Opals. The black Opal is vibrating to strengthen the receiving cells, and the white Opal is vibrating to strengthen the transmitting nerves.

The other basic property of the brain is blood. The brain receives its nourishment of food and oxygen from the blood. The Fire Opal corresponds to blood in the brain. In discussing a healthy brain, or the effects of the Opal on health, are we speaking of the psychological health of the brain, or of tissue health? We know they cannot be separated. If there were some physical or tissue damage in the brain, the Opal would be helpful in its physical presence. If the damage were to the psyche of the brain, the Opal would serve the same purpose. As the brain is the central switchboard of the whole body, it therefore effects every physical part. Enough emphasis cannot be placed on the value of this mysterious set of factors.

Psychic Strengths

Considering the correspondence of the Opal to the brain, it is important to trace the origin of the word *brain*. The Greek word was *bregma*, meaning "forehead." The origin of the word *Opal* is also Greek, *ophthalmos*, meaning "eye." In esoteric and metaphysical terms, the "third eye" is directly behind the forehead. The "third eye" is the eye that sees without really seeing. When we mean "I understand," we say, "I see." Constant references throughout history to the "evil eye" (meaning the ability to cause action simply by casting a ray of invisible power from the eye) or the "third eye," which we cannot see but know is there, or to the word *invisible* are perfect clues to the vibration spectrum of the Opal.

A person who has reached a state of awareness and has a desire to communicate with another by brain waves alone can accomplish it. That is transmitting. To be even more productive in the New Age, the brain wave must be changed into a different vibration known as alpha, in which the completed circuit is "receiving." There are many messages being sent out.

The secret we must learn at this point is to distinguish which messages are helpful in communicating and which must be filtered out. The Opal can be used in meditation as a "facilitator" and simultaneously as a filter. The most desirable information to be received is, of course, directly from the Universal Originator of all thought. The information that needs to be filtered out is negative or destructive, malfunctioning energy that behaves much like a cancer cell. Once it is allowed a resting place, it begins to agitate the other cells (ideas) around it, finally attaching itself to them and actually devouring them. In this manner negative emotions or thought patterns destroy positive brain waves.

The Opal has a dual message in its coded vibration. Unless it is known and understood, it will not be helpful to a novice. The transmitting and receiving process is one message. The filtering of information is the other.

The messages to be received from the Opal through meditative use are directly related to a fuller understanding of the inner workings of the spirit and of humankind. The psychic properties in this sense go further than sending and receiving information. To imply that the Opal is simply a transmitter-receiver is to overlook the basic visual quality—the great variation of fiery, flashing colors. This corresponds to its many and varied attributes in the psychic realm.

OPAL MEDITATION

The Opal, transmitting Neptune's ray-waves, is a great help in reflexology's treatment of the whole body by working on the feet.

An individual who has reached a state of awareness and who has a desire to communicate with another by transmitting brain waves can accomplish this. To be even more productive in the New Age, the brain wave must be changed into an alpha vibration in which the completed circuit is received as well as transmitting.

The Opal can be used in meditation as a facilitator for transmitting and simultaneously as a filter for receiving. Having a dual message in its coded vibration, it will not be helpful to a novice unless this is known and understood.

The messages to be received from the Opal through meditative work are directly related to a fuller understanding of the inner workings of the spirit. These include the ability to:

1. Activate psychic centers
2. Promote understanding
3. Make channeling possible
4. Heal brain and foot disorders
5. Discourage addictions

Method

Lie down on the floor on your back. Hold the Opal in your palm and gaze at it for one full minute.

Place the Opal against the . . .

SOLAR PLEXUS (near waist): Cover with palm, repeat seven times . . . "This Opal is vibrating to activate my psychic centers."

HEART: Cover with palm, repeat seven times . . . "This Opal is vibrating to power my center of understanding."

FOREHEAD ("third eye"): Cover with palm, repeat seven times . . . "This Opal is vibrating so that I may receive and channel information from above."

The Black Ray Source Unknown

ONYX

The origin of the black ray is not known at this time. Occult teachers throughout history have theorized that the black ray surrounds the physical world in order to screen out and prevent any part of the physical from returning to its source of spirit until perfecting itself through experience, test, and trial.

Described by all religions, the Christian word for this blackness is "chaos," from the Greek word meaning "formless, infinite space." In the Hebrew Cabala it is called the "negative existence." There are many other names in other religions, but the interpretation is the same, namely, when manifestation at all levels ceases to be.

Where this ray enters the body is also unknown, but the

area most likely would be one of the centers of the head. The black ray can be explained as a destroyer through absorption. Death is usually described as black or darkness, creating a negative connotation for us. When regarded as only the time preceding light, as in the night, we no longer fear the black ray.

The blackness of sleep and death are only short periods without the light. Many people having experienced near-death have described it as a blinding light as they pass through darkness into another level of awareness.

ONYX

CHEMICAL COMPOSITION: SiO_2 (silicon dioxide)
CRYSTAL SYSTEM: hexagonal (trigonal)
BLACK RAY
PLANET: Unknown
POWER CENTER UNKNOWN
HEALTH FACTOR: Absorption, immune system
PSYCHIC QUALITIES: Information gathering

General Science

Onyx is the layered version of Agate, specifically in black and white layers. These layers are mostly even and parallel, white above black. If the layers are brown and white, it is called Sardonyx; red and white is "Cornelian-onyx." If Chalcedony is found black only in color, it is called Onyx. There is also a type of marble found in Mexico, the U.S., South America, and North Africa that is incorrectly called Onyx-marble. It is of a different chemical makeup (calcite-aragonite). Do not confuse Onyx with marble.

Since all of the locations where Agate is found have already been listed, and the historical notes have been recorded in the Agate chapter, this treatise will concentrate on the psychic properties of black-white Onyx.

History, Myth, and Magic

Onyx rings have been used for thousands of years as seal rings, engraved with coats of arms or initials. The raised images are the white layer, while the background is the black. The reverse is to carve down through the white into the black, which is called intaglio. Finding the black-white-layer Onyx in nature is rare. The best samples are from Brazil and Argentina.

In an effort to produce this effect, regular Agate is dyed black and bleached in streaks, or slices of dyed black are glued together with white and called doublets. Do not be fooled.

Healing Secrets

The Onyx directly affects the immune system. It is working on the black ray from the cosmos. James Sturzaker gives this ray the character of conservation and absorption. The black ray may appear to be dull or lackluster. However, it is made sharp and clear through the allegiance of the white.

This black ray controls the two opposites in our bodies that protect us from contagious diseases and infectious bacteria. The killer corpuscles that attack foreign germs are directed by the black ray. The blood-strengthening corpuscles are affected by the same polarity.

If a person has disease in the body, or will be exposed to foreign bacteria, the use of an Onyx will encourage balance in red-white cells and strenghten the immune system.

Psychic Strengths

The parallel between the physical and the spiritual level of the black-ray vibration is "absorption." If it is diseased physically, mentally, or spiritually, the black ray can absorb and transmute it.

The psychic quality of the stone Onyx could well be used by research scientists, especially those now aggressively studying Acquired Immunodeficiency Syndrome (AIDS), which is a new infectious disease in our civilization. The Onyx would not only help the victims of this as yet incurable, deadly disease, but it could help the scientists to gather information leading to its extinction. As the black ray would absorb the disease, it would also throw a bright light on the immune system that could lead to the cure of other infectious or cancerous killers.

The lighter side of the Onyx is its ability to locate lost objects by detecting their vibrations. It is a very physical stone. Missing objects, or missing persons, can be detected if the Onyx is focused in meditation. It is especially helpful if used as a detector in psychometry with some physical piece that has been with the lost person or item.

In any case, the Onyx can do nothing by itself. It must be worn and used daily in meditation.

ONYX MEDITATION

If a person has disease in the body, or will be exposed to foreign bacteria, the use of an Onyx will encourage a balance between red and white cells, thereby strengthening the immune system.

Onyx could well be used by research scientists studying Acquired Immunodeficiency Syndrome (AIDS).

It can do nothing by itself, however. It must be worn and used daily in meditation.

The Onyx:

1. Is a listening stone, gathering information
2. Helps to find lost articles
3. Assists physical strength and overcomes weakness
4. Balances the hemoglobin

Method

Lie down on the floor on your back. Hold the Onyx in your palm and gaze at it for one full minute.

Place the Onyx against the . . .

SOLAR PLEXUS (near waist): Cover with palm, repeat seven times . . . "This Onyx is vibrating to gather all information."

HEART: Cover with palm, repeat seven times . . . "This Onyx is vibrating to increase my physical strength."

FOREHEAD ("third eye"): Cover with palm, repeat seven times . . . "This Onyx is vibrating to help me find lost articles."

Sugilite
THE NEW CRYSTAL

This chapter on the Sugilite crystal I have held apart from the other categories. Because it has come to us so recently, I believe it is in perfect timing for the enormous changes in our social and economic structure. This crystal will be a basic tool to aid us in making the transformation on a global and personal level. (For more information on coming changes, see chapter 4, The Coming of the New Age.)

SUGILITE

CHEMICAL COMPOSITION: (K,Na) (Na Fe^{3+}) 2(Li Fe^{3+}) Sil2°30
BURGUNDY AND VIOLET RAYS
PLANETS: PLUTO and MERCURY

General Science

The first find of Sugilite was made in 1944 by Professor Kenichi Sugi, a distinguished petrologist after whom the gem was named. Discovered in the Iwagi Islet in southwest Japan, Sugilite measures 6½ on the Mohs' scale of hardness from 1 to 10. Sugilite is a deep purple to magenta colored stone.

When the first gem quality Sugilite was discovered in the Kalahari Desert, it was marketed in small amounts of fine jewelry. When it was introduced in the early 1980s it was called Royal Azel. Other sources from South Africa have called it Lavulite because of its deep lavender color.

The name Sugilite has been officially approved by the Commission of New Mineral Names of the International Mineralogical Association.

The type of deposits are crystalline beds or veins. The chunks resemble Lapis Lazuli in appearance of opaque stone. Sugilite is finding its way to the United States constantly.

The Planetary Connection

I believe the discovery of the planet Pluto in our solar system in 1930 caused the discovery of Sugilite.

The rampage of four world wars began shortly after Pluto arrived. Chaos precedes transformation. The wars, which appeared as tragedy in our short sight, actually moved the lagging countries ahead, spread worldwide resources, brain, and human potential into every primitive area.

The color rays that are transmitted through Sugilite are the violet and burgundy. The planets are Mercury and Pluto.

After two years of doing the meditation exercise of placing it on my solar plexus, heart, and forehead every day, I believe I have received some parts of the vibration messages.

I have mounted two polished pieces with a silver moon Opal in a pendant that I wear daily over my heart. I have a rough piece to hold, bathe, and take to bed.

My clients have also reported their reactions after a 28-day trial, using this method.

The vibrations from the planets Pluto and Mercury seem to be transmitted by the Sugilite to help take us back in time to transform what we are presently experiencing into understanding our needs on a primitive level. The Sugilite vibration transforms our hectic, high-tech lives into simple, basic, crystal geometry—a "planted seed sprouts above ground and is transformed in plant" type of recollection. Understanding where we have lived in other worlds or other types of bodies in this world is an awakening. It transforms and grounds us to emotionally feeling and mentally knowing that everything in the Universe, and indeed in our lives, is progressing slowly but surely in the intended direction.

I find that very deep in the primeval Emotional Body there is a place that we as humans living in a fast changing and evolving society can retreat to be healed. We can calm trauma we experience when we come here to Earth in the physical form. I believe that the spirit or soul exists throughout various types of life on other planets and other Universes. We have experienced lives on the Earth in the dense physical forms of crystal, plant, and animal existence. I believe in the Universal Law of constant evolution and constant transformation. The greatest turbulence, chaos, and destruction occurs within the crystal as heat and pressure fuse atoms, minerals, and molecules into a perfectly gorgeous orderly geometrical pattern. THAT is transformation. The seed in the ground is ripped and torn asunder as the sprout bursts forth to become the beautiful plant. The lovely smooth egg is cracked, split, and irreparably destroyed as the fluffy chick emerges. These are transformations we have all personally experienced on our primordial Earth home.

Healing Secrets

When terrific turbulence or extreme change is taking its toll on the Mental and Emotional Body, meditation with a Sugilite can relieve fear. Physical symptoms are expressed by the adrenal and pituitary glands in shock. This is commonly called the "fight or flight syndrome." The heart speeds up, the stomach feels uneasy, we lose our appetite, our hands perspire, yet feel cold. The blood vessels and surface muscles constrict, chemicals and hormones begin to pour into our system. These reactions are automatic. If we do not fight or run away, as the emotional body is demanding, all of these defense mechanisms hurt the physical body instead of helping it.

In daily life we are taught to control our Emotional Body, to be acceptable to others. We maintain a calm outward appearance, but while the Invisible bodies are in this destructive state we are going to experience various symptoms of pain.

Each person has a specific area of their physical body where the pain centralizes. Some experience migraine headaches, others have laryngitis, headcolds, or allergies. The most severe cases become crippling arthritis, cancer, or coronary attacks.

The Sugilite can cause an understanding to surface in our confused or anxious minds or emotions. Accepting that we have survived transformations over and over for millions of years and have constantly emerged on a higher and higher plane and level of evolution, will minimize any present trauma.

The Sugilite vibration can promote our connection to our own positive experiences in hundreds of life forms throughout the Universe. It can cause us to recollect the many past transformations in this life and how we had to surrender ourselves to be born again, on a higher level, every time. Surrender is not an act of failure, but an act of faith. To LET GO OF FEAR AND TO KNOW THAT LOVE IS CONSTANT IN THE UNIVERSE is the Sugilite message.

SUGILITE MEDITATION

Sugilite can relieve fear. It will calm the symptoms caused by overactive adrenal and pituitary glands due to stress. Symptoms include migraine headaches, laryngitis, head-colds, arthritis, cancer, or coronary attacks.

Sugilite can promote our recollections of past transformations in this life. It teaches the message that surrender is not an act of failure, but an act of faith. Let go of fear and know that love is constant in the universe.

Method

Lie down on the floor on your back, hold the Sugilite in your palm and gaze at it for one full minute.

Place the Sugilite against the . . .

SOLAR PLEXUS (near waist): Cover with palm, repeat seven times . . . "This Sugilite is vibrating to disintegrate my fears."

HEART: Cover with palm, repeat seven times . . . "This Sugilite reminds me to surrender everything to faith in my evolution."

FOREHEAD ("Third-eye"): Cover with palm, repeat seven times . . . "This Sugilite helps me recall all of my past successful transformations."

THE GOOD NEWS

Eight years ago during the time when our psychic energy group was holding our weekly meditations, other information came through me as I was speaking in trance. This was a detailed description of a future healing center to be "created" by thought, concentration, visualization. The name of the center was given as "Emerald City" and made reference to the metaphysical children's story *The Wizard of Oz*. Almost everyone in America and in many countries overseas has seen the motion picture starring Judy Garland.

I was told to take careful note of the design of the buildings, which used Buckminster Fuller's geodesic domes and pyramids. I was instructed this would be made physical only if I would "hold the vision."

I have held new moon, full moon, lunar eclipse, and solar eclipse gatherings, using visualization with large groups of like-minded friends. I have used the special cosmic energy of Halley's Comet and the powerful times of March 21 (spring equinox), June 21 (summer solstice), September 21 (autumn equinox), and December 21 (winter solstice) to bring our mind energies in focus on Emerald City's becoming real.

I have printed and mailed or given a small prospectus describing the project to thousands of interested people. The news has actually spread worldwide. Many people have sent me articles of other communities being planned with similar ideals. There may even be a few places in operation now, on a smaller scale.

Recently Shirley MacLaine has declared her intention to build such a center. Many of my friends encourage me to make contact with her.

I have always been a very active and constant worker. I have always been a builder. However, in this instruction I was told I must not attempt to make Emerald City happen in the traditional way. I was challenged to manifest the physical complex with the mind only. It would be a miracle.

Every miracle begins with a search for the invisible. I know Emerald City is already built in the invisible planes. It is time for the vision to materialize.

APPENDIX A

Crystal Structure

These are examples of the mathematical nature of the universe. These are only a few of the miraculous NATURAL formations of crystals born in our Mother Earth.

CLEAR QUARTZ	KUNZITE
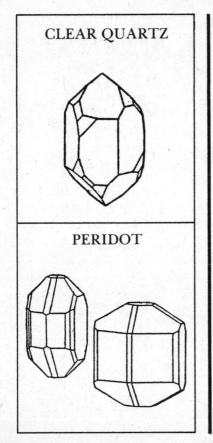	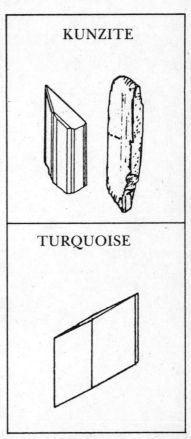
PERIDOT	TURQUOISE

OPAL

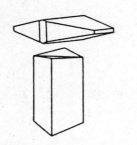

CORAL

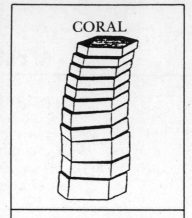

MALACHITE

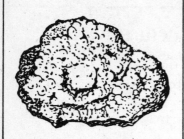

BLUE SAPPHIRE

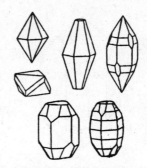

LAPIS LAZULI

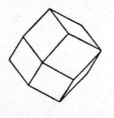

TOPAZ

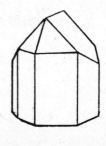

AQUAMARINE

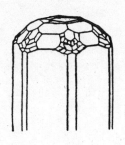

EMERALDS

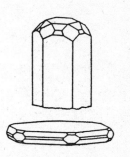

TOURMALINE

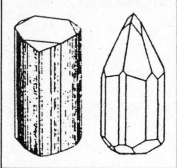

GREEN GARNET

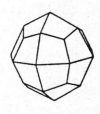

THE DIAMOND

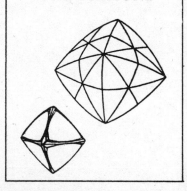

JADE—JADEITE

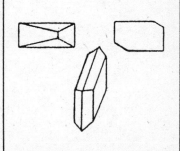

APPENDIX B

Emerald City

Dorothy, who wanted to go home, the tin man, who wanted a heart, the scarecrow, who wanted a brain, and the lion, who lacked courage, searched together for Emerald City. These four believed that the Wizard of Oz, who lived in Emerald City, had the power to grant their self-satisfying desires. After a long and arduous journey, this group discovered the Wizard was a nice person, but a fake. The moral of the story was twofold:

- No one could do it for them
- They already possessed within themselves the qualities they desired

THIS IS THE DRIVING MESSAGE OF THE NEW AGE EMERALD CITY!

Emerald City is conceived as a supportive community staffed by dedicated, talented, spiritually aware workers and teachers. Residence in the complex will be available for staff, but not required.

Vacation time for working people could be a healing time for the body, mind, and spirit. The nature communion available with outdoor activities, sun, and water would be enhanced by the most natural landscaping and design possible.

Emerald City is visualized as combining several successful ideas already working:

- Findhorn, a community for spiritual learning with

273

everyone working together in partnership with nature—located in Scotland.

- Disneyland where fantasy is made real and usable.
- La Costa, California, where people can vacation and temporarily experience the commune.
- The Golden Door in Southern California where the vacationer gets very individual treatment but is expected to experience group regimen.

Emerald City has no need to be separated by distance from the population. It can be isolated from worldly noise and distraction by its own environment. The flow of people will be directed by landscape design and grounds layout to give everyone a feeling of privacy in nature.

A distinct feeling of other-worldness will be promoted. The attitude of separation from the busy world will be included in the architecture and overall layout. Spaces for commercial offices, shops, and overnight accommodations will be camouflaged as imaginatively as possible. The basic aim is to provide a total environment for rejuvenation.

There may be certain areas designed to resemble the interior of a spaceship—or a primitive Indian village. Using the concepts of Walt Disney, Emerald City can bring all manner of joy and awakening to a group that may never find any other orthodox avenue to understanding. The subliminal messages, plus overt activities, must have a lasting effect upon any visitor.

Plans for Emerald City include a spiritual spa, retreat, reeducation, vacation, recreation, commercial shopping, restaurants, theater, new-age private school for children, and holistic new-age health care. The concept is unique in that it serves the local surrounding community as well as visitors from other states and countries.

Whether a person comes to attend self-realization classes, self-actualization seminars, metaphysical arts, the health and workout spa or to purchase personal vibration clothing or jewelry, the emphasis is on his or her growth.

Opportunities will be available for research in several areas, including medicine, human potential, nutrition, and gardening. Eventually food and decorative plants will all be cultivated on the premises.

Everyone connected in any way with Emerald City will have a deep desire for spiritual understanding. The basis for Emerald City's existence is to provide a better life for all concerned. Eventually there will be an Emerald City within every major city in the world.

Take a few minutes to meditate about where you fit into this marvelous concept.

Emerald City is a commercial enterprise—A "win-win" entity. If you are of like mind and desire to participate in this unique and dramatic metaphysical adventure—to assist in growing needs for endowments—you may contact me. Benefactors will be drawn to the development of Emerald City—a nucleus of realistic and objective metaphysicians are already fully committed to get Emerald City going.

FOR MORE SPECIFICS, SEND NAME AND ADDRESS TO: Brett Bravo
1903 South Catalina
Redondo Beach, CA 90277
(310) 373-5000

HERE'S TO YOUR PROSPEROUS FUTURE!!

BIBLIOGRAPHY

Books and Dissertations

Airola, Paquo. *The Total Approach to Health and Healing*. London: Emerson Press, 1963.

Amber, R.B. *Color Therapy: Healing with Color*. Calcutta: Firma LKM Private Ltd. 1964–1976.

Anderson, Mary. *Colour Healing: Chromotherapy & How It Works*. New York: Samuel Weiser, Inc. 1975.

Arem, Joel. *Gems and Jewelry*. New York: Bantam Books, 1983.

Arroyo, Stephen. *Astrology, Karma & Transformation*. Reno, Nevada: C.R.C.S. Publ., 1978.

Asimov, Isaac. *Understanding Physics: Light, Magnetism & Electricity*. New York: Signet, 1969.

Babbitt, Edwin, M.D. *Principles of Light & Color*. New York: Babbitt & Co. 1878. Reproduced by Health Research, Mokelumne Hill, 1956.

Baer, Randall N. & Vicki V. Baer. *The Crystal Connection*. San Francisco: Harper & Row, 1986.

Berne, Eric, M.D. *Sex in Human Relations*. New York: Simon & Schuster, 1970.

Birren, Faber. *Color Psychology and Color Therapy*. New Hyde Park: New York University Books, 1961.

Blavatsky, Mme. H.B. *The Secret Doctrine*. Wheaton, IL: Theosophical Pub. Original Publication: London, 1888.

277

Bryant, Page. *Crystals and Their Use*. Santa Fe, NM: Sun Pub., 1984.

Burka, Christa Faye. *Clearing Crystal Consciousness*. Albuquerque, NM: Brotherhood of Life, 1985.

Capra, Fritjof. *The Tao of Physics*. Berkeley, CA: Shambhala, 1975.

Cayce, Edgar. *Gems and Stones: Readings of Edgar Cayce*. Virginia Beach, VA: A.R.E. Press, 1976.

Chocron, Daya Sarai. *Healing with Crystals and Gemstones*. New York: Samuel Weiser, 1983.

Clark, Linda A. *The Ancient Art of Color Therapy*. Old Greenwich: The Devin-Adair Co., 1975.

Close, Stuart. *The Genius of Homoeopathy: Lectures and Essays on Homoeopathic Philosophy*. Calcutta: Haren & Bro., 1967.

Coddington, Mary. *In Search of the Healing Energy*. New York: Destiny Books, 1983.

Connelly, Dianne M. *Traditional Acupuncture: Law of Five Elements*. Colombia, MA: Center for Traditional Acupuncture, 1975.

Crow, W.B. *Precious Stones*. Wellingborough, England: The Aquarian Press, 1968.

Dana, James Dwight. *A System of Mineralogy*. London: Chapman and Hall, 1906.

Daya, Sarai Croshon. *Healing With Crystals & Gemstones*. NY: Samuel Weiser, 1983.

Diamond, John, M.D. *Your Body Doesn't Lie*. NY: Harper & Row, 1979.

Dinshah, Darias. *The Spectrochrome System*. Malaga, NJ: Dinshah Health Society, 1979.

Dinshah, P. Ghadiali. *Spectrochrommetry Encyclopedia: Measurement and Restoration of the Haman Radio-active and Radio-Emanative Equilibrium by Attuned Color Waves*. 3 vols. Malaga, N.J.: Spectrochrome Institute, 1933.

Donoghue, Michael, Editor. *Encyclopedia of Minerals & Gemstones*. London: Orbis Pub.

Finch, Elizabeth & W.J. *Photo-Chromotherapy*. Phoenix, AZ: Esoteric Publ., 1972.

Forley, Richard. *Rocks and Minerals*. London: Octopus Books.

Gallert, Mark, M.D. *New Light on Therapeutic Energies*. London: Jms. Clark & Co., 1966.

Goethe, Johann Wolfgang von. *Theory of Colors*. Trans. by Charles Eastlake. Cambridge, MA and London: The MIT Press, 1970. First Publication London, 1840.

Govinda, Lama Anagarika. *Foundations of Tibetan Mysticism*. New York: Sam Weisner, 1972.

Hanoka, N.S. M.D. *The Advantages of Healing by Visible Spectrum Therapy*. India: Bharti Asso. Pub., 1957.

Heindel, Max. *Occult Principles of Health and Healing* Oceanside, CA: Rosicrucian Fellowship Press, 1938.

―――. *Rosicrucian Cosmo-Conception*. Oceanside, CA: Rosicrucian Fellowship Press, 1909.

―――. *Message of the Stars*. Oceanside, CA: Rosicrucian Fellowship Press, 1973.

Heline, Corinne. *Healing and Regeneration Through Color*. Marina del Ray, CA: DeVorss, 1944.

Hutchison, Robert. *The Search for Our Beginnings*. New York: Oxford University Press, 1983.

Kapoor, Dr. Gouri Shanker. *Gems & Astrology*. New Delhi: Ranjan Pub., 1985.

LaForest, Sandra & Virginia MacIvor. *Vibrations*. New York: Samuel Weiser, 1979.

Leakey, Richard E. and Roger Lewin. *Origins*. New York: E.P. Dutton, 1977

Lewis, Thomas A. *Planet Earth Gemstones*. Chicago: Time-Life Books, 1983.

Littlefield, Charles W., M.D. *Man, Minerals and Masters*. Albuquerque, N.M.: Sun Publishing, 1980.

Lowen, Alexander, M.D. *Bioenergetics*. New York: Coward, McCann & Geoghegan, 1975.

Ludzia, Leo. *Life Force*. St. Paul, MN: Llewellyn Publications, 1987.

Lüscher, Dr. Max. *The Lüscher Color Test*. Translated and Edited by Ian Scott. New York: Random House, 1983. Original Publication: Basel, Switzerland, 1948.

Mann, W. Edward. *Orgone, Reich and Eros*. New York: Simon & Schuster, 1973.

Matteson, Barbara J. *Mystic Minerals*. Seattle, WA: Cosmic Resources, 1985.

Moody, Raymond A. Jr. M.D. *Life After Life*. New York: Bantam, 1976.

Myers, F.W.H. *Human Personality and Its Survival of Bodily Death*. New Hyde Park, NY: University Books, 1961.

Olsen, Dr. Edward and David Techter. *Rocks, Minerals and Gems*. Northbrook, IL: Hubbard Scientific Co., 1970.

Ott, John, Phd. *Light & Health*. New York: Simon & Schuster, 1973.

Ott, John, Ph.D. *Light, Radiation and You*. Old Greenwich, CT: Devin Adair, 1982.

Paracelsus. *Paracelsus Selected Writings*. Edited by Jolande Jacobi, translated by Norbert Guterman. Princeton, NJ: Princeton Univ. Press, 1973.

Pelletier, Kenneth R. *Mind as Healer, Mind as Slayer*. New York: Dell Publishing, 1977.

Ponder, Catherine. *The Healing Secret of the Ages*. West Nyack, NY: Parker Pub., 1967.

Rabonewitz, Ra. *Cosmic Crystals*. Wellingborough, England: Turnstone Press Ltd, 1983.

Rabonewitz, Ra. *Cosmic Crystal Spiral*. Longmead, England: Element Books, 1986.

Raphael, Katrina. *Crystal Enlightenment*. New York: Aurora Press, 1985.

————. *Crystal Healing*. New York: Aurora Press. 1987.

Rea, John D., *Healing and Quartz Crystals Vol. 1*. Boulder, CO: Two Trees, 1986.

Sauer, Jules Roger. *Brazil, Paradise of Gemstones*. Hamburg: Grafica Editoria, 1982.

Schumann, Walter. *Gemstones of the World*. New York: Sterling Pub., 1977.

Scott, Miners, Editor. *A Spiritual Approach to Male-Female Relations*. Wheaton, IL: Theosophical Publ., 1984.

Silby, Uma. *The Complete Crystal Guidebook*. New York: Bantam Books: 1986.

Sinkankas, John. *Minerology*. NY: Van Nostrand Reinhold Co., 1964.

Smith, Michael G. *Crystal Power*. St. Paul, MN: Llewellyn Publ., 1985.

Snyder, Robert. *Buckminster Fuller*. New York: St. Martin's Press, 1980.

Stein, Dianne. *Women's Book of Healing*. St. Paul, MN: Llewellyn Publications, 1987.

Sturzaker, James. *The Twelve Rays*. New York: Samuel Weiser, 1976.

Sykes, Egerton & Donnelly, Ignacias. *Atlantis, The Antediluvian World*. New York: Harper & Row, 1949.

Techter, David. *Stereogram of Rocks, Minerals & Gems*. Hubbard Scientific IL 1970.

Thomas, Lewis, M.D. *The Medusa and the Snail*. New York: Viking Press, 1979.

Walker, Dael. *The Crystal Book*. Sunol, CA: The Crystal Col, 1983.

Ancient Manuscripts

Bhaktivedanta, Swami Prabhupada. *Srimad Bhagavatam* from the original Sanskrit text. Bombay, India, 1972.

Braun, Johann. "Vestitus Sacerdotim Hebraeorum," Ancient Manuscript on Microfilm, Berlin Public Library, West Berlin, Germany. 1378.

Dawood, N.J., translator. *The Koran*. NY: Viking Penguin Inc., 1956.

Ghadiali, Dinsha P. (known as Dinsha). *Spectrochrometry Encyclopedia*: Measurement and Restoration of the Human Radio-active and Radio Emanative Equilibrium by Attuned Color Waves. 3 Vols. Malaga, NJ: Spectrochrome Institute, 1933.

Gimma, Giaccinto. "Della Storia Naturale delle Gemme," Ancient Manuscript on Microfilm, Vatican Library, Rome, Italy. 1730.

Hohnemann, Samuel. "Organon of Medicine." Ancient Manuscript on Microfilm, Microfilm Library, West Berlin, Germany. 1842.

Lamsa, George M., translator. *The Holy Bible from Ancient Eastern Manuscripts*. Nashville, TN: A.J. Holman Co., 1933.

Marbodus. "De Lapidibus." Ancient Manuscript on Microfilm, Vatican Library, Rome, Italy. 1531.

Megenberg, Konrad von. "Buch der Natur." Ancient Manuscript on Microfilm, National Museum, Berlin, West Germany. 1861.

Finot. "Les Lapidaires Indiens", Mineral Collection, Sorbonne, Paris. 1896.

Trismegistus, Hermes. "Writings on the Divine Pymander." Ancient Manuscripts on Microfilm, National Library, Museum University, Athens, Greece. 375 A.D.

Magazine Articles

Heydon, Daniel. "The Impact of Uranus on the World and You, Part II," *Dell Horoscope*, May 1984.

Tauraso, Nicola Michael, M.D. "Light on Your Health," Wholistic Life Magazine, 1984.